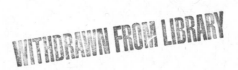
Exposed Science

Exposed Science

GENES, THE ENVIRONMENT, AND THE POLITICS OF POPULATION HEALTH

SARA SHOSTAK

UNIVERSITY OF CALIFORNIA PRESS
Berkeley   Los Angeles   London

University of California Press, one of the most distinguished university presses in the United States, enriches lives around the world by advancing scholarship in the humanities, social sciences, and natural sciences. Its activities are supported by the UC Press Foundation and by philanthropic contributions from individuals and institutions. For more information, visit www.ucpress.edu.

University of California Press
Berkeley and Los Angeles, California

University of California Press, Ltd.
London, England

Library of Congress Cataloging-in-Publication Data

Shostak, Sara.
  Exposed science : genes, the environment, and the politics of population health/Sara Shostak.
    pages cm
  Includes bibliographical references.
  ISBN 978-0-520-27517-1—ISBN 978-0-520-27518-8
  1. Environmental health—Political aspects.   2. Pollution—Environmental aspects.   3. Health risk assessment.   I. Title.
  RA566.S56   2013
  613'.1—dc23
                                        2012035261

Manufactured in the United States of America
22 21 20 19 18 17 16 15 14 13
10 9 8 7 6 5 4 3 2 1

In keeping with a commitment to support environmentally responsible and sustainable printing practices, UC Press has printed this book on Rolland Enviro100, a 100% post-consumer fiber paper that is FSC certified, deinked, processed chlorine-free, and manufactured with renewable biogas energy. It is acid-free and EcoLogo certified.

For my family, and especially for my mother,
Myra Shostak, of blessed memory.
"For love is strong as death . . ." (Song of Songs)

Contents

Acknowledgments

Whenever I stop to consider how many people's generosity, wisdom, and support have helped me bring this project to fruition, I am both awestruck and profoundly grateful. I hope that these acknowledgments go some small way toward expressing my appreciation.

To the respondents who participated in this research, I owe a great debt. The generosity with which many busy people met my requests for their time, their stories, their aspirations, and their insights made this research possible. Moreover, the passion, humor, and consideration expressed in these meetings made conducting the research a true pleasure. I am grateful to Richard Sharp, for bringing me into the Program in Environmental Health Ethics and Policy at the National Institute of Environmental Health Sciences (NIEHS) as an intern in 2002, and to Ben Van Houten, who generously agreed to be my science mentor that summer.

The first round of data collection and analysis was guided by my wonderful dissertation advisor, Adele Clarke, to whom I am forever indebted for introducing me to science and technology studies (STS) and qualitative research methods; this project would not have happened without her. Meeting with Adele and the members of my committee—Howard Pinderhughes, Paul Rabinow, and Sharon Kaufman—was always both helpful and a delight. I am grateful for the guidance, friendship, and inspiration of each of these scholars.

The second round of data collection was facilitated by the DeWitt Stetten, Jr., Memorial Fellowship in the History of Biomedical Sciences and Technology at the Office of NIH History. In addition to the collegial environment of the Office of NIH History, I benefited tremendously from the opportunity to continue conducting interviews and observation at the NIEHS. I especially thank Kenneth Olden, Raymond Tennant, Samuel Wilson, and Mary Wolfe for their support of my fellowship.

The Robert Wood Johnson Foundation's (RWJ) Health and Society Scholars Program at Columbia University was a transformative experience. I am a better—and braver—sociologist thanks to the mentorship of Peter Bearman. I learned important lessons about how to be an advocate for my ideas from Bruce Link. I am grateful to David Rosner, Ezra Susser, and Ruth Ottman, each of whom, in his or her own way, has helped me to better understand public health and to crystallize my commitment to it. I also thank Peter Bearman, Molly Martin, and Jeremy Freese for helping me "think with" genetics in new and productive ways.

Since 2006, I have had the great fortune to be on the faculty at Brandeis University. I thank my colleagues in sociology for their support and enthusiasm for my research and teaching. I am especially indebted to Peter Conrad for bringing to his role as my faculty mentor both wisdom and good cheer. Teaching the Approaches to Social Research proseminar with Wendy Cadge and David Cunningham has been a treat, as well as a valuable opportunity to think critically about knowledge production in the social sciences. I am grateful also to the faculty in the Health: Science, Society, and Policy (HSSP) and Environmental Studies Programs for the opportunity to create innovative learning experiences at the intersection of disciplines. I consider myself extremely fortunate to teach and learn from the many wonderful students at Brandeis, whose commitments to social justice inspire and sustain my own.

I gratefully acknowledge the support of the National Science Foundation Program in Science, Technology, and Society for a Doctoral Dissertation Improvement Grant. I am thankful also for generous funding from the UC Toxic Substances Research and Teaching Program, the UC Berkeley Program in Social Studies of Science and Technology, the Agency for Health Care Research and Quality, and the Graduate Division of UCSF. I thank the UC Humanities Research Institute both for a White Fellowship in Medicine and the Humanities and for the opportunity to participate in the Resident Research Group on Health and Place. When I arrived at Columbia University, this research was further supported with a seed grant from the RWJ Health & Society Scholars Program. Completing and illustrating the manuscript were made possible thanks to a grant from Brandeis University's Theodore and Jane Norman Fund for Faculty Research.

I delight in the collective and collaborative nature of sociological research and am thankful for the many excellent comments I've received on this work. The analysis was certainly improved by the insights of participants at meetings of the American Sociological Association, the Society for Social Studies of Science, and the RJW Foundation Health & Society Scholars Program. Likewise, I have benefited from the opportunity to give papers at Brown University (at varying times to the Contested Illness Research Group, the Program in Science and Technology Studies, and the Race and Genomics Lecture Series), the Boston University Center for Philosophy and History of Science, the Harvard University Science and Technology Studies Circle, the National Institutes of Health, the Stanford Center for Biomedical Ethics, the Department of Sociology and the Science and Justice Working Group at UC Santa Cruz, and the Departments of Sociology and of Anthropology, History, and Social Medicine at UC San Francisco.

For their time and consideration in reading drafts of chapters—and, in some instances, the entire manuscript—I offer my heartfelt thanks to Rene Almeling, Peter Bearman, Debbie Becher, Jason Beckfield, Ruha Benjamin, Catherine Bliss, Phil Brown, Wendy Cadge, Monica Casper, Peter Conrad, David Cunningham, Scott Frickel, Micah Kleit, Sabrina McCormick, Alondra Nelson, Aaron Panofsky, David Pellow, Jenny Reardon,

Sarah Richardson, David Rosner, Natasha Schull, Janet Shim, Stefan Timmermans, Jocelyn Viterna, and Peter Wissoker. For helping me navigate my way through the writings of Pierre Bourdieu, I thank Aaron Panofsky, Rebecca Lave, and Catherine Bliss. I am grateful to Phil Brown for suggesting that I write what became the Afterword, and for being a role model for scholars interested in the intersections between sociology, health, and the environment. I really could not ask for better colleagues and am happy to count so many of these scholars as my friends.

I am indebted to Phil Brown and David Rosner for directing me to Hannah Love, the editor for health at the University of California Press. Hannah guided the manuscript through the review process with a mix of intelligence and grace that was a true blessing for a new author. I was privileged, then, to work with Naomi Schneider during the process of revising and bringing the manuscript to press. I thank Chris Lura and Francisco Reinking for their skillful project management.

No words are adequate to express my appreciation to my friends for the love, cheerleading, solace, and great company that they have provided in the decade it took me to complete this project. I trust that you know who you are when I say thank you for taking long walks with me, inviting me to stay with you (in California each winter, in New York year-round), indulging my need for adventures (especially by the ocean), showing up (sometimes across great distances) without my even asking, offering your home as a writing retreat (and writing there with me), sharing summer veggies (thank you to Waltham Fields Community Farm for the veggies themselves), sitting with me in silence (even for a week at a time), going out with me to hear music (as well as being the source of that music), encouraging me to bike and to read and to garden and to cook, and, in so many ways, reminding me of all that is beautiful in the world. Two very young people brought especial gifts: Jackson and Arabella. Thank you for singing to my Mom—and me—during difficult moments.

Finally, I humbly offer boundless love and gratitude to my family. To my father, Peter, whose unwavering faith in me and my abilities set me on the right path and, when needed, helped me keep moving forward. To Eli and Erin, whom I would choose to have by my side in any situation, and to Delia Jane, whose presence brings such joy. To Matt, who gave me safe harbor when I needed it most and seems to be able to make me laugh in any situation. A Kauany, minha linda enteada. And to my mother, Myra, whose unending strength, ability to love, capacity for amazement, and commitment to "turn toward gratitude" made me who I am and continue to inspire me every day.

Introduction

In the spring of 2000, a two-year-old girl named Sunday Abek was treated at a New Hampshire hospital emergency room for a low-grade fever and vomiting. Because her throat culture was positive for strep, the doctors sent her home with a prescription for an antibiotic. Her condition worsened, and three weeks later Sunday was admitted to the hospital, where she fell into a coma. Two days later, she died. The cause of her death was lead poisoning.

Originally from Sudan, Sunday's family had recently moved to the United States from an Egyptian refugee camp, where she had lived for most of her brief life. She was poisoned, however, by lead in her family's home in an apartment building in Manchester, New Hampshire. Following her death, testing at the apartment revealed that the porch, where Sunday played, was covered with peeling, flaking paint.[1] Window wells in the apartment were contaminated with lead dust. At the time of her death, Sunday's blood lead level was 391 µg/dL (micrograms of lead per deciliter of blood), nearly 40 times higher than the threshold at which a child is considered to have lead poisoning.[2]

Less than a century ago, severe lead poisoning of infants and children was a major public health challenge (Markowitz & Rosner 2002; Rabin 1989). Children are more susceptible to lead poisoning than adults for numerous reasons. Per kilogram of body weight, children drink more fluids, eat more food, breathe more air; they also have a larger skin surface in proportion to their body volume. Children absorb a larger fraction of ingested lead than do adults, and they are more greatly affected by absorbed lead. Children's behaviors—crawling, putting things in their mouths, playing outdoors—also increase their risk of lead exposure.[3] However, Sunday was the first child to die of lead poisoning in the United States in over a decade (Lord 2001).

Lead poisoning in children became a preventable disease as a result of decades of research and advocacy by environmental health scientists, progressive social reformers, and policy makers (Markowitz & Rosner 2002; Sellers 1997). In the United States, primary prevention—that is, preventing exposure—is at the center of efforts to protect children from the harmful effects of lead.[4] Public policy has played an especially prominent role. In 1973, the Environmental Protection Agency (EPA) mandated the phaseout of lead in gasoline.[5] In 1977, the Consumer Products Safety Commission (CPSC) limited the lead in most paints. Similarly, the United States has banned the use of lead in food containers, children's toys, and municipal water systems. Together, these regulations resulted in a 78% reduction in human exposure to lead between 1976 and 1991 in the United States, as measured in blood lead levels (Pirkle et al. 1994; 1998). This is one of the major public health success stories of the last quarter century (Grosse et al. 2002).

Despite these successes, thousands of U.S. children, especially low-income and minority children, are exposed to harmful levels of lead each year.[6] As blood lead levels have fallen nationally, *disparities* in lead exposure and lead poisoning have increased. According to the Centers for Disease Control and Prevention (CDC), lead-based paint in older housing, along with the contaminated dust and soil it generates, remains the most widespread and dangerous high-dose source of lead exposure for young children. From 1991 to 1994, 16% of low-income children living in older housing had elevated blood lead levels, compared to 4.4% of all children (CDC 1997). Likewise, low-income children living in older housing have more than a thirty-fold greater prevalence of elevated blood lead levels compared to middle-income children in newer housing (Pirkle et al. 1998). Between 1997 and 2001, of the children reported with confirmed elevated blood lead levels, approximately 60% were African American (CDC 2003). The apartment building where Sunday Abek's family lived was built in 1910 and, at the time of her death, was home to families who had immigrated recently from Kosovo, Sudan, Rwanda, and Zimbabwe (Daniel 2001).[7]

Simply put, although children share biological susceptibility to lead, they are not equally at risk for lead poisoning. Rather, vulnerability to lead poisoning is socially determined. Because they are more likely to live in older houses, low-income and minority children are more likely to be exposed to lead and to suffer from lead poisoning (Lanphear et al. 1998). Recognizing the social factors that make low- income children more susceptible to lead poisoning, the President's Task Force on Environmental Health Risks and Safety Risks to Children[8] has called for targeting federal grants to control and remediate lead hazards in low-income housing and expanding blood lead screening and follow-up services for at-risk children, especially Medicaid-eligible children.

At the same time that the environmental health scientists on the President's Task Force were calling for programs and policies that would address the social factors that make children susceptible to the harmful effects of lead exposure, their colleagues had begun to develop a very different way of conceptualizing how we become vulnerable to lead. In October of 2000, researchers at the Johns Hopkins School of Public Health published the results of a study on lead conducted in Korea[9] that focused on variations in a person's genetic makeup, which, in part, determine how lead is handled by the body (Schwartz et al. 2000). The study found that people who carry specific variants of two genes had significantly higher blood, bone, and chelatable[10] lead levels. This project was funded by the National Institute of Environmental Health Sciences' (NIEHS) Environmental Genome Project, a high-profile research initiative that sought to identify genetic variations that modify the body's response to environmental exposures, thereby making some people more vulnerable to the harmful effects of toxic substances. The scientists who worked on this study are world-renowned experts in environmental and occupational health. The lead author is particularly well-known for his research on the health effects of cumulative lead exposure. As a result of this work, he has suggested that the measures currently used to regulate occupational exposure to lead (e.g., blood lead levels) are an insufficient basis for assessing risk because they reflect only recent—rather than lifetime—lead exposures; such research has clear and important policy implications. And, these respected environmental health scientists—and public policy advocates—were among many whose research, in the early 1990s, turned to the question of genetic susceptibility to environmental exposures. This book asks what motivated scientists to study gene-environment interaction and explores the consequences of environmental health research that focuses inside the human body and at the molecular level.

LEAD INSIDE THE HUMAN BODY?

At the center of this book are the interlinked puzzles of *why* and *how* environmental health scientists rallied around research on gene-environment interaction. To frame these puzzles narrowly—again by focusing on the case of lead—we might ask:

- Given that so much is known about the harmful effects of lead, the social factors that put children at risk of lead poisoning, and the demonstrated though partial successes of policy approaches to reducing lead exposure in the U.S. population, why would the NIEHS prioritize research on the genetics of lead absorption?

- What do scientists believe can be learned about how to prevent lead poisoning by looking deep inside the human body, at the molecular level?

- Given the lead industry's history of calling into question children's genetic susceptibilities and behaviors as a means of denying the harmful health effects of lead,[11] why would scientists committed to public health study gene-lead interactions?

- Is there any reason to think that knowledge about gene-environment interaction can help to protect low-income and minority children, who are most at risk of lead poisoning?

- Conversely, by focusing attention at the molecular level, might research on gene-environment interaction obscure, however unintentionally, the social, political, and economic factors that make low-income and minority children particularly susceptible to lead poisoning?

To answer these questions, I conducted interviews with more than eighty environmental health scientists, policy makers, and environmental justice activists. I was a participant-observer in research laboratories, at scientific symposia, and at meetings of activists. I undertook a comprehensive review of scientists' publications.[12] In brief, I found that environmental health scientists offer three broad types of answers, not only in regard to research on lead in particular, but, more generally, on research on gene-environment interaction.

First, environmental health scientists emphasize the ongoing challenges posed to environmental health research insofar as it is used as a basis for regulating industries that produce toxic substances.[13] For example, one environmental health scientist noted that, although "we have known about the health effects of lead for two thousand years" and clearly can reduce these effects without knowledge of gene-lead interactions, given how "politicized" environmental regulation is, having data about molecular genetic mechanisms "does help make the point" (Interview S50). Related, scientists frame research on gene-environment interaction as a solution to a variety of sources of uncertainty in their research. For regulators who are "constantly fighting an uphill battle with economic forces that would rather preserve the status quo" (Interview S50), any source of perceived scientific uncertainty makes the regulations based on environmental health research vulnerable to legal challenge.[14] Indeed, as documented both by historians and by regulatory scientists, "manufacturing uncertainty" has itself become a "big business" as companies seek to prevent, delay, and overturn regulation (Michaels 2008: 46). Challenging the relevance and/or reliability of the science supporting regulatory decisions is a key strategy of "merchants of doubt" (Oreskes and Conway 2010).[15] According to a prominent environmental health scientist, the contentious dynamics between "industry" and "environmental protection" have become the "drumbeat" to which the field works (Interview S27). Scientists express hope, therefore, that molecular genetic and genomic technologies will make their research findings more robust, especially in the context of risk assessment and regulation (Olden & Wilson 2000).

In a second set of answers, environmental health scientists point to the rising power of the idea that all human disease is a genetic phenomenon. To the extent that scientists, policy makers, and the general public assume that genes are primary determinants of human health and illness,[16] even when research seeks to evaluate disparities in lead poisoning that are most likely "explained by socioeconomic differences, social differences, and exposure differences that vary by the neighborhoods in which people live," it must also assess genetic influences: "[I]f you want to . . . convince people that it's *not* genes, you've got to measure genes" (Interview S11). Thus, scientists believe that research on gene-environment interaction may play a role in protecting the jurisdiction (Abbott 1988) of the environmental health sciences, that is, investigation into how the environment affects human health.

Scientists' third set of answers also centers on jurisdictional concerns, highlighting the possibility that research on gene-environment interaction might generate not only a more robust basis for regulation, but also new biomedical markets for their research. Traditionally, environmental health science has contributed to environmental health risk assessment and regulation; it serves as the empirical basis for public policies that seek to reduce environmentally associated disease at the population level. In regard to its potential to improve public policy, scientists suggest that research on individual genetic variation in susceptibility to environmental hazards demonstrates that existing regulations provide insufficient protection and require revision: "[W]hat it does in that

situation is it allows you to say, if we're going to protect children . . .
then it's not enough to protect the average kid. You've got to protect this
more [genetically] vulnerable group" (Interview S06). At the same time,
research on gene-environment interaction has the potential to foster a
"a more biomedical environmental health" (Interview S20), in which
environmental health science would inform behavioral and clinical interventions for reducing the harmful health effects of environmental exposures; thus, scientists envision going beyond the "status quo" of "we
tell the EPA and FDA and OSHA [that a substance is harmful] and they
regulate" (Olden, Oral History Interview July 2004). For example, identifying high-risk individuals might contribute to the development of so-
called "lifestyle prescriptions" to minimize the risks of exposure or to
new pharmaceutical interventions to prevent harmful consequences of
exposure (Olden, Guthrie, & Newton 2001). The NIEHS leadership sees
new behavioral and biomedical strategies as especially important for
substances like lead because "it's going to be a long time before we get
many of these things out of our environment" (Olden, Oral History Interview July 2004). Further, such an individualized, biomedical approach
is well aligned with neoliberal public health policy regimes (Peterson &
Lupton 1996).

TOWARD A SOCIOLOGY OF THE ENVIRONMENTAL HEALTH SCIENCES

Each of these answers points to a part of the story told in this book. However, these explanations make sense only within a broader analysis of the
field of the environmental health sciences. As such, this book takes the
ascendance of gene-environment interaction within the environmental
health sciences as an analytic lever[17] that reveals important dimensions
of the structure of the field of environmental health science; its central
institutions; the commitments, practices, and strategies of those working
within it; and how this shapes what we know about—and how we seek to
govern—the relationships between the environment and human health.
The central argument is that scientists' perceptions of and responses to

the *structural vulnerabilities* of the field of environmental health sciences have both intended and unintended consequences for what we know about the *somatic vulnerabilities of our bodies* to environmental exposures.

In crafting this analysis, I draw on several different theoretical frameworks, each of which supports inquiry into a different aspect of environmental health research and its consequences. This theoretical tool kit enables me to ask questions about the structure of the environmental health sciences as a *field*, to examine the relationships between key *institutions*, to conceptualize environmental health scientists as *skilled social actors*, and to investigate the *biopolitical effects* of their recent strategies.[18] To be clear, my goal in this book is not to extend a given theoretical framework (see Burawoy 1999), but rather to solve an empirical puzzle. Consequently, I use these perspectives to help me identify, describe, and fit together a variety of puzzle pieces. In the following chapters, these theoretical tools appear as "points of departure" and as "a means for generating new questions" (Lamont 2012).

Fields Theory

To begin, I draw on fields theory, an analytic approach (Martin 2003: 24) that highlights the importance of analyzing the forces and struggles within fields (Bourdieu 1996, 1998, 2004).[19] Recent writing on *strategic action fields* directs analytic attention to four aspects of a field: (1) a diffuse understanding of what is going on in the field, that is, what is at stake (Bourdieu & Wacquant 1992); (2) sets of actors in the field who possess more or less power; (3) a set of shared understandings about the rules of the field, or how "the game" is legitimately played; (4) an interpretive frame that individual and collective actors use to make sense of activity within the field (Fligstein & McAdam 2011: 4).

In this particular case, a big part of what is at stake is the ability to make legitimate and robust claims about the causes of environmental health and illness.[20] As such, among the questions explored in the following analysis are:

- What are the rules of the field? Who has the technical capacity and the social power to speak and act legitimately in this domain (Bourdieu 1975: 19)? What kinds of capital govern status within the field?

- What hierarchies exist among actors in the field? Who are the dominant players? That is, which actors have managed to impose a definition of science that says that its highest realization "consists in having, being, doing, what they have, are, and do . . . " (Bourdieu 2004: 63)? What options are available to scientists whose research is seen as inferior? How might actors endeavor to define good science in ways that will benefit them by increasing the value of the *kind* of science they do?

- What is the subjective structure, or *habitus*, that social actors within the field acquire through participation in it (Bourdieu 1996)? [21] What "possibilities and impossibilities" are thereby "offered to their dispositions" (Bourdieu 2004: 36)?

Recent writing on strategic action fields has emphasized also the importance of the broader field environment, or what I call an arena.[22] As noted by Fligstein and McAdam, "virtually all of the work on fields focuses only on the internal workings of these orders, depicting them as largely self-contained, autonomous worlds." However, fields do not exist in a vacuum; relationships and boundaries with other fields are often powerful parts of a field's developmental history (Fligstein & McAdam 2012: 59). Insofar as we fail to attend to the ties that link fields to each other—and to the arenas (or broader field environment) in which they are located—we constrain our ability to understand field dynamics, "including the potential for conflict and change in any given field" (Fligstein & McAdam 2011:8). It is especially important to understand the relationships between a given field and that subset of state and nonstate fields on which it routinely is exposed. [23]

A central consideration is the extent to which the field is independent from demands—or shocks—from actors and/or events outside the field. Against the assumption that scientific fields are always "autonomous and isolated," with changes in science driven primarily by dynamics internal to the field (Albert & Kleinman 2011; 267; Mialet 2003; see also Bourdieu 1975: 29), I seek to investigate empirically conflicts regarding the autonomy and legitimacy of specific forms of knowledge production.[24] In so doing, I demonstrate that in the environmental health arena, scientific claims, the struggle for scientific authority, and ongoing political and economic concerns have become deeply intertwined.

Second, my work draws on the insights of institutional theory regarding how fields are constituted and may be reconstituted through patterns of institutional interactions and relations.[25] Neoinstitutional theory also focuses on fields but conceives of them more broadly as "those organizations that, in the aggregate, constitute a recognized area of institutional life: key suppliers, resource and product consumers, regulatory agencies, and other agencies that produce similar services and products" (DiMaggio & Powell 1983: 148). Neoinstitutional theory posits that the structure of fields is a consequence of the requirements and demands of the state, the structure of the professions, and competition for resources, political power, and institutional legitimacy. Most broadly, an institutional approach to the sociology of science attends to the "rules and routines, organizations, and resource distributions that shape knowledge production systems" (Frickel & Moore 2006: 7).

Historically, scholars in this tradition also have asked questions about two different, if often interrelated, forms of institutional change. First, scholars have investigated the processes through which institutions come to resemble each other, identifying mechanisms of isomorphic change such as coercion (a consequence of political influence and problems of legitimacy), mimesis (by which institutions copy each other in an effort to manage uncertainty), and norms that are established and transmitted through professional networks (Schneiberg & Clemens 2006). Second, and related, they have asked questions about the diffusion of innovations, behavioral strategies and organizational structures, and their adoption (Strang & Soule 1998: 268). Research on diffusion points to the importance of structural mechanisms, such as social networks and reference groups (Burt 1987; Granovetter 1973; Simmons, Dobbin, & Garrett 2008; Strang & Soule 1998). At the same time, sociologists describe diffusion as a deeply cultural process; for example, the cultural understanding that organizations or institutions belong to a common social category may provide the basis for a tie between them (Strang & Meyer 1993: 490–492). As we will see, both the *competition* and the *connections* between NIH institutes, such as the National Cancer Institute (NCI) and NIEHS, and between regulatory agencies, especially the Food and Drug Administration (FDA) and EPA, have motivated, constrained, enabled, and been reshaped by the diffusion of molecular genetic and genomic techniques. [26]

Viewed through these theoretical lenses—and, as highlighted by the scientists whom I interviewed—the environmental health sciences faced myriad challenges in the waning decades of the twentieth century. I detail these challenges in the following chapters. In brief, they include the relative lack of autonomy of the environmental health sciences as a field,[27] ongoing challenges to and critiques of environmental epidemiology and toxicology in controversies over risk assessment and regulation, the rising power of genetic (versus all other) explanations for human health and illness, and growing concern that specific institutions of environmental health research—including the NIEHS and the National Toxicology Program (NTP)—were losing status, funding, and political support. My argument in this book is that research on gene-environment interaction, with its focus inside the human body and at the molecular level, has been compelling to environmental health scientists precisely insofar as it offers a diverse array of strategies for meeting these challenges.[28]

Strategies and Consequences

Environmental health scientists had choices about how they responded to these challenges, and the decision to take up research on gene-environment interaction was not without risks. I ask "How did environmental health scientists, as "skilled social actors" (Fligstein 2001), perceive, evaluate, and pursue this particular strategy for strengthening their field, garnering resources for their institutions, protecting their professional jurisdiction, and doing important and meaningful scientific research, as they understand it?[29] To answer this question, the subsequent chapters take up also the following topics:

- What motivated environmental health scientists to make gene-environment interaction a defining focus of their research?

- How did environmental health scientists build a coalition around the idea that understanding gene-environment interaction is integral to disease prevention and public health? What identities or stories were at play in constructing this coalition?

- How have environmental health scientists articulated the relevance of gene-environment interactions in the context of a field that historically has oriented primarily on public policy rather than on biomedical interventions?

- In what ways have scientists adapted molecular genetic and genomic technologies, developed originally to study the health of individuals, to answer questions about how environmental exposures affect population health?

- How did advocates for research on gene-environment interaction in the environmental health sciences mobilize support for this view of the future of the environmental health sciences?

Answering these questions requires a careful consideration of the history of the environmental health sciences, especially environmental epidemiology and toxicology, and the relationships among biomedicine, public health, and public policy. [30] Therefore, although the phenomena that I seek to explain are decidedly contemporary, my analysis is and must be deeply historical.[31] The historical accounts highlighted in this book come from archival data, scientists' written and oral reflections on the trajectories of research in their individual laboratories and/or field, and the work of historians of science and medicine. History is important to understanding actor's strategies, which vary under different conditions of power and uncertainty; moreover, as will be seen, such strategies have drawn extensively on existing rules, resources, understandings and controversies regarding the warrants of particular fields, institutions, and professions (Fligstein 2001: 106). In crafting this aspect of the analysis, I draw on a relatively loose understanding of *path dependence*, that is, the insight that key decisions at earlier points in time produce outcomes that set history on a course from which it is often is difficult to return (Katznelson 2003: 290).[32] At the same time, I am interested in how the past can be a source of creativity as well as constraint; history may not only foreclose options but "may also lead to and shape the switch points confronted by later generations, drawing fault-lines along which later crises erupt and creating options for new solutions" (Haydu 1998: 357).

Lastly, I consider the consequences of these transformations for how we understand and intervene in the relationships among human bodies, the environment, and health and illness. Specifically, I argue that examining how environmental health scientists and policy makers have taken up, modified, and advocated for research on gene-environment interaction provides an important means of understanding what we know and don't know about relationships about our bodies, the environment, and human health and illness.

In making this argument, I draw on contemporary writings on biopolitics and coproduction. *Biopolitics* refers broadly to "all the specific strategies and contestations over problematizations of collective human vitality, morbidity and mortality" (Rabinow & Rosee 2006: 195–217; see also Foucault 1978/1990). Today, three elements constitute biopolitics: "[k]nowledge of vital life processes, power relations that take humans as living beings as their object, and the modes of subjectivation through which subjects work on themselves qua living beings" (Rabinow & Rose 2006). The central insight of *coproduction* is that our ways of knowing the world are inextricable from controversies regarding how to best live in it (Jasanoff 2004). To understand biopolitics, then, one must examine not only knowledge production, but also the politics of institutions, the making of identities, and their relationships to each other (Epstein 2007). In the context of environmental health, these perspectives highlight the importance of tracing the relationships among knowledge production in the environmental health sciences, the governance of environmental risks to human health, the identification of individual and groups at risk, and the development of notions of the ethics and responsibilities of such persons. When stabilized in relationship to each other, these elements produce a biopolitical paradigm, that is, a "framework of ideas, standards, formal procedures, and unarticulated understandings that specify how concerns about health, medicine, and the body are made the simultaneous focus of biomedicine and state policy" (Epstein 2007: 17). Although we may not be aware of it, the biopolitical paradigm of the environmental health sciences profoundly shapes how we live today.

Chicago Bans Bottles with BPA plastic.[33] *San Francisco Passes Cellphone Radiation Law.*[34] *Bottle Maker to Stop Using Plastic Linked to Health Concerns.*[35] *Ground Zero Workers Reach Deal over Claims.*[36] Current newspaper headlines highlight the many ways that the environmental health sciences enter into our daily lives, determining not only what technologies and products we use, but also what we know about their effects on our health.[37] Federal regulatory agencies, such as the EPA and FDA, and their counterparts at the state and local levels, use the results of environmental health research to determine the methods and extent to which they will regulate the emission of industrial chemicals into our communities and whether products containing specific chemicals should remain on the shelves of grocery and drug stores. Industries use data from environmental health research to decide what combinations of chemicals they will use to produce consumer products, as well as to justify their decisions when they are challenged by regulators or activists. In the courts, environmental health science contributes to decisions about whether people who have been exposed to an environmental contaminant should receive compensation for its effects on their bodies or on the bodies of their children. At the same time, as consumers, we increasingly are called upon to use information from environmental health research to make personal choices about the potential risks of the water we drink ("That Tap Water Is Legal but May Be Unhealthy"[38]), the food we eat ("High Mercury Levels Are Found in Tuna Sushi"[39]), and the products we use on our bodies and in our homes ("Should You Worry About the Chemicals in Your Makeup?"[40]) (Szasz 2007).

Given the critical role of environmental health research in modern life, social scientists have paid remarkably little attention to the fields, institutions, social actors, and practices most central to the production of contemporary environmental health science.[41] To date, research has tended to focus on the social life of the *products* of environmental health science, as when specific research on the health effects of a chemical are challenged by environmental health activists (Allen 2003; Brown 2007; Corburn 2005), denied by industry (Brandt 2007; Markowitz & Rosner 2002; Oreskes & Conway 2010; Proctor 1995), or (re)interpreted by legislators (Jasanoff 1990; Keller 2009), rather than examining the scientific research practices and institutional contexts through which such claims come into being. These studies of community-based environmental health controversies and challenges to environmental regulation provide rich analyses of the contentious politics of the environmental health arena. What remains understudied is how contemporary environmental health scientists make choices about the foci and methods of their research, seek to transform processes of risk assessment and regulation, and protect the legitimacy of their field, all in the context of these ongoing political and legal challenges.

GENE-ENVIRONMENT INTERACTION: FROM AN "ANNOYING DETAIL" TO "OUR MANTRA"

The ascendance of gene-environment interaction as a way of understanding how the environment affects human health, its institutionalization[42] in environmental health research and policy making, and the responses and critiques of environmental justice activists provide the substantive foci of this book.

In the past three decades, environmental health scientists have redefined human genetic variation from an "annoying detail" to a "central determinant of risk" in research on environmental illness (Hattis 1996; see also Puga et al. 1996). By the early 1990s, the NIEHS had made gene-environment interaction its "mantra" (Olden, Oral History Interview July 2004). The NIEHS's investment in research on gene-environment interaction was instantiated in "flag raising initiatives" (Interview S27), such as the Environmental Genome Project, the National Center for Toxicogenomics, and the Toxicogenomics Research Consortium, and in increased extramural funding for university-based efforts to develop the subfield of molecular epidemiology. Gene-environment interaction is now at the center of collaborations between the NIEHS and the National Human Genome Research Institute (NHGRI), such as the Genes, Environment, and Health Initiative (GEI), a multimillion-dollar project launched in 2006 to identify genetic predispositions and improve the measurement of environmental exposures associated with common diseases, such as asthma, autism, and diabetes (NIEHS 2006).[43] NIEHS administrators contend that these initiatives have transformed the standing of their institute:

So, we started [the genomics initiatives] . . . and the National Institute of Environmental Health Sciences has become a major player at the National Institutes of Health. It used to be, quite frankly, that they didn't see us as important to the mission of the National Institutes of Health, to protecting public health. But now we are a major part of the Institutes—we are integrated with the National Cancer Institute, the National Human Genome Research Institute—and they see how important our work is for public health (Field Notes, NIH December 2001).

As described in the following pages, the genomics initiatives have also transformed profoundly the research practices of many environmental health scientists.

To date, environmental health scientists have established two broad ways of studying gene-environment interaction. First, scientists seek to identify genetic susceptibilities that make some people more vulnerable to being harmed by environmental exposures. In this framing of gene-environment interaction, scientists acknowledge the harmful effects of environmental contaminants, but genetic variations in individuals' responses to them are the crucial problem to be explained. Second, scientists examine how environmental chemicals affect human genetic material, whether by causing DNA damage (e.g., mutations) or by altering gene expression (e.g., epigenetics). In this framing of gene-environment interaction, scientists acknowledge human genetic variability, but the effects of environmental exposures are the crucial problem to be explained. Although environmental health scientists have long been interested in how environmental pollutants damage DNA (Frickel 2004), they describe the broad integration of molecular genetic and genomic techniques as a "revolution" in their field (Field Notes, NIEHS 2002).

In recent years, this molecular revolution has redefined what it means to do environmental health research in the United States. As a leading molecular epidemiologist[44] recalled, in the early 1990s, when he first arrived in the department of environmental health sciences at a prestigious school of public health, his colleagues challenged the molecular biological focus of his work:

There was a lot of reluctance to accept the concept that molecular biology had something to say in environmental health. There were many, many older faculty people who weren't even willing to accept that. [They said] . . . "This is not right. This is bullshit. You are not studying environmental health."

However, he continued, over time "those people started losing their funding and we started getting our funding. And then the emphasis shifted . . . now we really have created a large group of [scientists studying] molecular biology in the department" (Interview S20). Departments of environmental health science across the country now teach and conduct molecular genetic and genetic research as part of their standard coursework and in the context of interdepartmental programs.[45] Environmental health scientists advocate for research on gene-environment interaction by claiming that protecting population health requires investigation of "how the environment operates at the molecular level."[46]

The development of molecular genetic and genomic technologies and practices within the environmental health sciences has not gone unnoticed by other key actors in the arena of environmental health politics. The EPA and FDA have launched partnerships with the NIH and NTP to explore the application of molecular techniques in risk assessment and regulation. One such initiative, Tox21, endeavors to create a system of environmental risk assessment and regulation that replaces whole animal bioassays with *in vitro* methods that will evaluate the effects of chemicals by examining changes in cell lines (NRC 2007b: 1).[47] The chemical industry has taken a keen interest in these developments; in 2001, the International Council of Chemical Associations held a workshop and subsequently promulgated their recommendations for "best practices" for emerging "-omics" technologies[48] (Henry et al. 2002). Environmental health and justice activists have responded to the emergence of molecular genetic and genomic techniques both with curiosity about their potential for enhancing advocacy efforts and with intense criticism of what they see as the limitations and dangers of looking for the causes of human health and illness through a molecular genetic lens.

The critiques of EJ activists highlight the population health implications of environmental health research. A critical issue is whether environmental inequalities are an underlying cause of pervasive health disparities in the United States (Brulle & Pellow 2006; Evans and Kantrowitz 2002). There is evidence that income is often directly related to environmental quality; likewise, there is evidence that poor environmental quality is related to multiple physical and psychological health outcomes (Evans & Kantrowitz 2002: 324). These associations hold for exposure to a wide range of suboptimal environmental conditions (e.g., hazardous wastes and other toxins, ambient and indoor air pollutants, water quality, ambient noise, residential crowding, housing quality, educational facilities, work environments, and neighborhood conditions). Thus, it is possible that "the accumulation of exposure to multiple, suboptimal physical conditions rather than any singular environmental exposure" may accounts for the inverse relationship between income and a wide variety of health outcomes (Evans & Kantrowitz 2002: 304; see also Williams et al. 2010). Consequently, researchers have suggested that integrating data on environmental inequality and its health impacts into the existing research on health disparities is critical to efforts to understand the causes and identify solutions to the ongoing problem of health disparities between demographic groups in the United States (Brulle & Pellow 2006). These concerns about health inequalities have shaped the meanings of research on gene-environment interaction in the environmental health sciences, as well as the efforts of scientists and regulators to build consensus around the potential applications of genomic knowledge in risk assessment.

NOT JUST GENETICIZATION

In its analysis of the ascendance of research on gene-environment interaction in the environmental health sciences, this book contributes also to recent efforts to push social scientific analysis of molecular genetics and genomics beyond the geneticization thesis. *Geneticization* refers to "an ongoing process by which differences between individuals are reduced to their DNA codes" (Lippmann 1991: 19). Fundamentally, this approach asks us to consider whether and how genes are understood to be the primary cause of health, illness, and other forms of human variation. The concept of geneticization has been at the center of much social scientific analysis, where it often serves as connotative shorthand for a number of interlocking concerns about the myriad potential negative social implications of genetics; however, research suggests that the consequences of molecular genetics and genomics are more complex and contingent (Freese & Shostak 2009). Moreover, I contend that if, following the lead of the geneticization thesis, our analyses focus primarily on the extent to which scientists continue to study environmental causes of variation in human health and social outcomes, we miss the opportunity to observe profound changes in how genes, environments, and human bodies are conceptualized and operationalized in scientific research.

Therefore, in contrast to the geneticization thesis, I draw on the work of social theorists and historians of science to conceptualize the ascendance of research on gene-environment interaction as the *molecularization* of the environmental health sciences (de Chadarevian & Kamminga 1998; Kay 1993; Rose 2007). The molecular vision of life visualizes, operationalizes, and seeks to act upon life itself—including genes, environments, bodily variations and behaviors—at the submicroscopic level (Kay 1993). The molecularization of biology and medicine began in the 1910s, bringing profound changes in understandings of the causes and appropriate treatment of disease. Broadly speaking, contemporary uses of pharmaceuticals, vitamins, and hormones in biomedicine have their origin in the molecular vision of human health and illness (de Chadarevian and Kamminga 1998: 4; Sturdy 1998). However, even as some disciplines, such as biology, have been extensively molecularized, others, including the environmental health sciences, continued to conduct many of their operations well above the molecular level. For example, while specific domains of toxicology have made use of molecular biological technologies and concepts (Frickel 2004), many of the most important indices of toxicity used in toxicological risk assessments exist at what scientists describe as the "phenomenological" level: body weight, organ weight, level of activity, tumors, and death.[49] In environmental epidemiology, researchers historically focused on the relationships between exposures, disease, and death at the population level, without looking inside the "black box of the human body" (Interview S04).

Molecularization has met with myriad challenges in the context of environmental health research. Analytically, these challenges make the environmental health sciences an advantageous case for observing the social processes through which molecularization is accomplished. First, molecularizing environmental health research has required that scientists find ways to operationalize gene-environment interaction in work objects (Casper 1998), technologies, and experimental systems relevant to environmental health research. As belied by their names—e.g., environmental response genes, molecular biomarkers—most often, these new objects and practices are hybrid forms that combine more traditional objects with new materials or techniques. The following chapters describe the development of these new ways of doing environmental health research. At the same time, this is a deeply historical analysis, attending particularly to how new techniques extend previous research practices, are shaped by institutional concerns, and seek to address the structural vulnerabilities of the field.

Second, and related, much research in the environmental health sciences is directed toward applications in environmental health risk assessment, regulation, and policy making. Assessing whether a chemical causes mutations in DNA has been a required part of the registration of new chemicals since the passage of the Toxic Substances Control Act in 1976 (Frickel 2004). However, the regulation of the ambient environment depends rather on measurements of chemicals in the air, water, and soil; historically, it has not taken gene-environment interaction into account. Related, the gold standard of toxicological testing relies on the thirteen-week and two-year rodent bioassays and other whole animal studies (NTP 2002). Consequently, even as environmental health scientists argue that molecular genetic and genomic techniques will improve their contributions to environmental regulation, they have had to develop what I call *technologies of translation* as a means of articulating new modes of knowledge production within established regulatory processes.

Third, and again in contrast to many other domains of research in the life sciences, molecularization requires that environmental health scientists develop strategies for conceptualizing and measuring not just the human body, but the *environment* at the molecular level. Such strategies have emerged as a site of contention between scientists and environmental justice activists. In particular, activists question the appropriateness of molecular measures, given the extensive evidence of race- and class-based inequalities in environmental exposures (Brulle & Pellow 2006; Evans& Kantrowitz 2002). Many activists are concerned that social structural factors that put poor people and people of color at increased risk of environmental exposure will be obfuscated, however inadvertently, as research on molecular genetic research recasts the environment as something best understood and measured at the molecular level.

Simply put, the environmental health sciences provide an intriguing vantage point for studying the consequences of genetics precisely because the *environment* is their jurisdictional focus. In fact, some environmental health scientists position their research on gene-environment interaction as a corrective to the Human Genome Project's genocentric view of human health and illness: "[G]enocentric views reflect a fundamental misunderstanding of the disease process, and have led to unrealistic expectations and disappointment" (Olden & White 2005: 721). In contrast to genocentrism, environmental health scientists contend that research on gene-environment interaction is the key to explaining when and how genetic variations shape human health and illness: "Differences in our genetic makeup certainly influence our risks of developing various illnesses. . . . We only have to look at family medical histories to know that is true. *But whether a genetic predisposition actually makes a person sick depends on the interaction between genes and the environment*" (NIEHS 2006; see also Schwartz & Collins 2007).

Sociologists have expressed skepticism about the extent to which scientific research on gene-environment interaction actually represents an alternative to geneticization. Some have suggested that research on gene-environment interaction generates merely a narrative of "enlightened geneticization," which privileges genetic explanations and minimizes the effect of environmental factors, even while acknowledging that they play a role in human health and illness (Hedgecoe 2001). Others note that media coverage of research on gene-environment interaction selectively emphasizes genes and largely ignores environmental causes (Horwitz 2005).

My analysis shifts the focus, however, to the question of how different kinds of research on gene-environment interaction conceptualize and measure genes, environments, and their effects on human bodies. This allows us to see that at stake in this research is not only the question of whether genes or the environment cause human health and illness. Rather, I demonstrate that, by conceptualizing and measuring the environment at the molecular level, research on gene-environment interaction has profound consequences for how we understand the environment and how it affects our health.

ONE "Toxicology Is a Political Science"

In September 2007, an array of prominent environmental health scientists and activists was called to testify before Congress. Seated before the Domestic Policy Subcommittee of the House of Representative's Committee on Oversight and Government Reform were Samuel Wilson, then acting Director of the National Institute of Environmental Health Sciences (NIEHS), George Lucier, former Director of the National Toxicology Program (NTP), Lynn Goldman, a professor of environmental health science at the Johns Hopkins University School of Public Health, Peggy Shepard, the Executive Director of the EJ group West Harlem Environmental Action (WEACT), and Stefani Hines, a member of the National Advisory Environmental Health Sciences Council (NAEHSC).[1] The question before them was no less than whether the NIEHS was fulfilling its public health mission. Specifically under scrutiny was "a new set of research priorities" at the NIEHS, which had been implemented by its recently departed Director, David Schwartz.[2] The chairman of the subcommittee opened the hearing with two questions: "At what cost has come Dr. Schwartz's new direction for the NIEHS?" and "Should the new NIEHS research directions and priorities . . . continue?" (US GPO 2007: 2).

Particularly at stake in the hearing was the boundary between biomedicine, with its focus on curing disease in individuals, and public health, with its focus on population-based disease prevention. In fact, the focal concern of the subcommittee was whether the NIEHS was becoming *too biomedical* in its orientation and thereby failing to meet its public health mandate. In his opening comments, the subcommittee chair expressed concern about the shifting of "significant resources toward research that was clinical in nature and which focused on discoveries that would contribute to treating or curing disease once a patient was already afflicted" (US GPO 2007: 1). In advance of this hearing, the staff of the subcommittee had "performed its own analysis of the NIEHS' new research direction and priorities" and reached the conclusion that the public health focus of the NIEHS was being replaced with "programs of a clinical nature" (US GPO 2007: 2).

During the hearing, the speakers used a series of contrasts to distinguish the NIEHS and the NTP in particular, as well as the environmental health sciences more broadly, from the clinical focus of most biomedical research. To begin, in contrast to research that focuses on clinical treatments, *the environmental health sciences focus on disease prevention:* "NIEHS is the only institute with a primary mission of public health, rather than clinical medicine . . . " (US GPO 2007: 69). In contrast to research that is oriented to the development of new drugs or medical treatments, *the environmental health sciences inform public policy,* "mak[ing] major impacts on human health through research translation to public policy, not to the bedside" (US GPO 2007: 69). In contrast to research that is individually oriented, *the environmental health sciences contribute to protecting the health of the population,* serving as "the source of key information regarding the health impacts of pollution . . . used daily in setting protective federal, state, and local policies, in arguing for the protection of children, the elderly, and our communities" (US GPO 2007: 77). In contrast to research that is defined by a specific disease or organ, *the environmental health sciences investigate environmental exposures which affect multiple bodily systems and are associated with myriad diseases:* "Every disease has an environmental component, thus NIEHS's responsibilities encompass all human diseases, rather than following the more common model of focus on a specific disease or organ system"[3] (US GPO 2007: 26). In contrast to research that can be accomplished in laboratory and clinical settings alone, *the environmental health sciences engage with affected communities and must consider their concerns:* "We must be productively linked to our constituents . . . to fulfill the promise of our mission" (US GPO 2007: 29). Again, the boundary between biomedicine and public health was a focal concern, as speakers emphasized that "prevention and environmental intervention represent the most effective and efficient ways to improve human health, and this core principle should not be lost in favor of technical, individually oriented medical solutions" (US GPO 2007: 72).

Given the preventive and public health focus of the scientists testifying before the panel, their comments regarding molecular genetics and genomics were quite striking. Genetics has most often been associated with exactly the technical, clinical, individually oriented biomedical approaches that scientists described as what the environmental health sciences are *not*. However, in their testimonies before Congress, these speakers highlighted molecular genetic approaches as a promising solution to the ongoing and seemingly intractable problems confronted by scientists who seek to explicate relationships between environments, human bodies, and health and illness. Repeatedly, in their description of the agenda of the NIEHS, they asserted powerfully the importance of "new opportunities in science" (US GPO 2007: 23), particularly in molecular genetics and genomics, for environmental health research. Goldman described the NIEHS as "positioned to harness the next generation of scientific advances, such as in molecular biology and genetics, in the service of advancing environmental health sciences" (US GPO 2007: 70). Wilson explicitly connected molecular genetics research to the public health mission of the NIEHS, stating, "Our understanding of how the environment operates *at the molecular level* can also provide insights on interventions and early markers for disease . . . " and emphasizing the importance of evaluating how "emerging technologies can be used to enhance public health prevention strategies" (US GPO 2007: 21, 28, emphasis added). Lucier highlighted the importance of "technological innovations and molecular biology" for the NTP. Likewise, Hines emphasized the importance of approaches that would "bring environmental health research out of the sidelines where it consists only of testing chemicals for toxicity into a more mainstream role where research would investigate how environmental agents contribute to specific diseases that impact public health on a large scale" (US GPO 2007: 79–80).

What can we learn from this hearing? First, the major institutions of environmental health research must answer to Congress for their actions. They are accountable, particularly, for their contributions to public health policy.[4] Their funding depends on meeting their missions and mandates, as understood by politicians in Congress. Second, and related, the environmental health sciences have defined themselves as being part of public health and in contrast to biomedicine. Indeed, the NIEHS consciously seeks to establish an identity as "the prevention Institute."[5] At the center of this distinction is the difference between *protecting health and preventing illness* using population-level interventions, such as environmental regulation, versus *treating disease* using individual clinical interventions, such as pharmaceuticals. Third, given their focus on population-level interventions, there has been a push within the environmental health sciences to engage with affected communities and to work collaboratively to address environmental concerns. Fourth, by 2007, leading environmental health scientists, standing in front of the legislative body that authorizes their funding, were making strong claims about the importance of molecular genetic techniques to their public health mission.

Explaining why and how molecular genetics became positioned as a critical component of environmental health research, regulation, and policy making is the central concern of this book. Toward that end, my goal in this chapter is to provide a map of the institutional actors in the U.S. environmental health arena and to introduce their relationships and key struggles. In so doing, I draw both on the comments made before Congress in 2007 and a broader sociological analysis.[6]

THE ENVIRONMENTAL HEALTH ARENA

Understanding Environmental Exposures

At the center of the environmental health arena are questions and controversies about whether specific environmental exposure poses a risk to human health and, if so, under what conditions (e.g., at what dose, via which routes of exposure, for whom, etc.) and how such risks are best controlled. Environmental health scientists and scientific institutions play a central role in this arena. In most instances, knowledge of environmental hazards is contingent upon "the 'sensory organs of science'—theories, experiments, measuring instruments—*in order to become visible or interpretable as hazards at all*" (Beck 1992: 27, emphasis in original). Chemicals in the settings where we live, work, and play, in what we eat, and in the products we use to care for our bodies, clean our homes, tend to our yards, and so on are often neither visible nor perceptible to the persons being exposed to them (Altman et al. 2008). Additionally, many toxic substances have a lengthy latency period before the effects of exposure emerge, and others may affect not the person exposed but her or his children (Schettler et al. 2000; Steingraber 2003). Consequently, people are exposed without their knowledge to combinations of chemicals as they move through their homes, workplaces, and communities. Moreover, although members of the public may fear, perceive, and even document evidence of suspected environmental hazards (Brown & Mikkelson 1994), the legitimate recognition of a risk requires the tools and practices of science: "So long as risks are not recognized scientifically, they do not exist—at least not legally, medically, technologically, or socially—and they are thus not prevented, treated or compensated for. No amount of collective moaning can change this, only science" (Beck 1992: 71).

This "scientization" has been challenged by environmental health activists, who argue that individuals and communities have important "lay knowledge" about environmental hazards (Corburn 2005) and should not be excluded from policy debates (Brown 2007: 19). There is some evidence that activists' challenges to the technical practices of environmental health science have created opportunities for new forms of knowledge production (Ottinger & Cohen 2011). Nonetheless, environmental health science remains the authoritative idiom for making claims about the effects of environmental exposures on human health. As we will see, science is therefore also the idiom in and through which controversies about the effects of environmental exposures and regulatory strategies take place.

Explaining the relationships among bodies, environmental exposures, and human health and illness is the primary focus of the sciences of environmental epidemiology and toxicology. *Epidemiology* is the study of "disease occurrence in human populations and the factors that influence these patterns" (Lillienfield & Stolley 1994: 3). Epidemiologists use a variety of study designs, all of which rely heavily on statistical techniques, for establishing and quantifying the relationships between exposure to risk factors and disease outcomes in human populations. Environmental epidemiologists focus particularly on the effects of exposures in the ambient environment (e.g., air, water, soil). *Toxicology* is "the study of the adverse effects of xenobiotics" (Gallo 1996: 3) and includes both the study of absorption, distribution, excretion, and biotransformation of such agents and the analysis of basic toxicological processes within specific organ systems. Although much toxicology is ultimately concerned with human health and illness, toxicologists rely heavily on animal models, in vitro bioassays, and laboratory research (Sellers 1997; NTP 2002). Epidemiology and toxicology are the "core sciences" of public health in the United States (Omenn 2000). Institutionally, academic departments of epidemiology and toxicology are located in schools of public health, where their faculties often staff multidisciplinary environmental health research centers.

The location of environmental health science within the context of public health has had profound implications for the work of environmental health scientists, shaping patterns of funding, defining markets for their research, and determining opportunity structures for employment. In contrast to much research in the contemporary life sciences, which is oriented to biomedical interventions such as new pharmaceuticals or devices, the primary consumers of environmental health research include risk assessors, regulators, and policy makers; there is no promise of a lucrative "magic bullet," or cure, to environmental exposures or their consequences. This dynamic was highlighted at the Congressional hearing, when the subcommittee chair noted ". . . a significant failure of the market system: there is little profit in prevention when compared to treatment" (US GPO 2007: 7). As such, there are few incentives for private sector investment in environmental health research, aside from that sponsored by companies seeking EPA or FDA approval for their products. As one environmental health scientist commented, " . . . in contrast to a lot of other biomedical research where there are opportunities to make money, to patent a new drug, to patent a new protein, [in the environmental health sciences] you're constantly fighting an uphill battle with economic forces that would rather preserve the status quo" (Interview S50).

The often adversarial and litigious nature of the regulatory process in the United States also has shaped research institutions, practices, and possibilities in the environmental health sciences. Indeed, environmental health research was institutionalized at the federal level, in part, as a response to dynamics of contention and litigation surrounding risk assessment by the federal regulatory agencies (Jasanoff 1990, 1995). In the late 1960s and early 1970s, the federal government invested in a massive expansion of research capacity designed to bolster risk assessment by generating new and better scientific practices and identifying omissions, mistakes, and biases in extant data, especially those obtained from nongovernmental sources, such as industry (Jasanoff 1990: 41).

The National Institute of Environmental Health Sciences

> The mission of the NIEHS is to support research
> to define the role of environmental agents in the
> initiation and progression of human disease.
> The goal is to use knowledge from this research
> to reduce adverse exposures and, thus, reduce
> preventable diseases and conditions.
> Testimony of Samuel Wilson (U.S. GPO 2007: 21)

In 1969, Congress established the NIEHS and mandated it to direct basic research on the effects of environmental factors on human health (RTI 1965; see also Frickel 2004). At the turn of the current century, the NIEHS mission was to "to reduce the burden of human illness and dysfunction from environmental causes."[7] The NIEHS is the only one of the National Institutes of Health (NIH) defined by an independent or etiologic variable—the environment—rather than a disease (e.g., National Cancer Institute, [NCI] National Institute of Neurological Disorders and Stroke [NINDS]), organ or organ system (e.g., National Eye Institute [NEI], National Heart, Lung, and Blood Institute [NHLBI]), or a population group and/or developmental process (e.g., National Institute for Child Health and Human Development [NICHD], National Institute on Aging [NIA]). In the words of a former scientific director of the NIEHS:

> the key thing about environmental agents is that they show no disease boundaries, so the same chemical that causes cancer could also cause pulmonary disease, Alzheimer's, etc. So one of the challenges to environmental health sciences is really to be able to look at all of these different diseases. We don't have the luxury of just studying cancer. Obviously we have a big institute that just studies cancer [NCI], but they [NIEHS] have to deal with cancer and neurodegenerative diseases, and pulmonary diseases and kidney diseases (Barrett, Oral History Interview February 2004).

NIEHS is also the only National Institute of Health not located in Bethesda, Maryland; rather, its campus is located in Research Triangle Park, North Carolina. The NIEHS contains both an intramural and an extramural division. In 2005, Congress authorized a budget for NIEHS of approximately $650 million.[8] The initiatives of the NIEHS include funding not only of intramural and extramural research programs, but also of programs focused on environmental justice and community-based participatory research, as well as a premier peer-reviewed environmental health science journal, *Environmental Health Perspectives*.[9]

The research agenda of the NIEHS is shaped not only by its orientation to public policy, but also by an awareness of the missions of the other National Institutes of Health. As I describe in the following chapters, in developing its genomics initiatives, NIEHS scientists were very aware of staying within their own "turf" or "territory" and not "overlapping" with those of other institutes (Interviews 27, 37). I was told repeatedly that the environment is what defines the jurisdiction of the NIEHS, especially in regard to other National Institutes of Health.

That being said, in the context of the contemporary life sciences, the term *environment* may refer to the cell (which is the environment of the gene), endogenous hormonal profiles (the internal environment of the cells, organs, etc.), indoor or outdoor ambient environments (the environment of the human body), diet and exercise, or stressful life situations. In recent years, environmental health scientists have appealed to broad conceptualizations of the environment and its relationships to public health as a means of integrating behavioral and lifestyle factors into their research.[10] In an oral history interview, in which he reflected on his years as the director of the NIEHS (1991–2005), Olden stated:

> *The environment was defined too narrowly when I got there* . . . It was chemical and physical, mostly chemical. They almost never thought of physical, but [when] they would, they thought of radiation. But I said, "you know, the environment's much more than that. *The environment is your lifestyle choice* . . . *it is diet, nutrition, certain pharmaceutical exposures, and things like poverty* . . . " And so we then expanded the definition and I see it being used more and more. More and more, our definition [is used] by everybody (July 2004, emphasis added).

The broader definition is used "by everybody" in part because of the success of NIEHS advocacy for it:

> There was an IOM [Institute of Medicine] Roundtable, around 1999, on environmental health that was the first workshop to endorse a broader definition. As a result, we felt empowered to embrace a wider definition and *we began to promote that wider definition.* For example, we worked with the surgeon general on the Healthy People 2010 document, which uses the wider definition of environmental health. And then it becomes a self fulfilling proposition, because we can, in turn, invoke the Healthy People 2010 definition . . . (Interview 27, emphasis added).

This expanded definition has been used to advance new foci at the NIEHS, including recent initiatives focused on obesity. As Olden explained:

> I wanted to be sure that when I went before Congress or you know and they found out that I was putting 10 to 20 million dollars into behavioral research, [they wouldn't say,] "Why are you doing that? That's not your mission." . . . As a matter of fact I just got the question from the Department [of Health and Human Services] about the Built Environment Conference. *So I had to give them the definition of the environment and then their objection went away* . . . (July 2004, emphasis added).

In other words, a broad definition of the environment provides a rationale for expanding the jurisdiction of the environmental health sciences: "This is great for the Institute. [It] allows us to expand our programs, our outreach" (Field Notes, NIEHS 2002).[11] In one such expansion, the Exposure Biology Program, which the NIEHS leads as part of the Genes, Environment, and Health Initiative (GEI), scientists are working on "the development of innovative technologies to measure environmental exposures, diet, physical activity, psychosocial stress, and addictive substances that contribute to the development of disease."[12] In fact, one of the first requests for applications issued by the program was for "Improved Measures of Diet and Physical Activity for the Genes and Environment Initiative."[13]

At the same time, the expansion of the definitions of the environment to include individual behavior—such as diet or physical activity or the use of addictive substances—represents a shift in the focus of environmental health research from largely involuntary exposures (e.g., chemicals in the air, water, and soil) to life-style choices which are, at least nominally, voluntary. Likewise, this may shift the focus of preventive strategies from public policy (e.g., environmental regulation) to individual behavior change.[14] As we will see, definitions of the environment in gene-environment interaction generally allow for both of these strategies; this, I argue, has been a factor in their success.

The National Toxicology Program

> The NTP . . . is considered a world class toxicology research and testing program and reports from the NTP are widely used around the world for strengthening the science base for regulatory decisions and for informing the public on health issues. Its role in disease prevention should not be minimized . . .
>
> Testimony of George Lucier (US GPO 2007: 59)

The NTP was founded in the wake of Congressional dissatisfaction with the performance of the NCI Bioassay Program, which had faltered in its efforts to expand testing programs as directed (and funded) by the National Cancer Act (Smith 1979). The NIEHS was given the "the lead role" in the NTP in 1978, by order of Health, Education, and Welfare secretary Joseph Califano. In 1981, the NCI Carcinogenesis Bioassay Program and, with it, many research scientists were transferred to the NIEHS. At that time, the NTP became a permanent activity of the Department of Health and Human Services (DHHS), charged with coordinating toxicological testing programs within the Department (Weisburger 1983).

Although the NTP contracts with facilities around the country, it resides on the NIEHS campus in Research Triangle Park, North Carolina. NIEHS scientists describe the mission of the NTP as "permeating" throughout the Institute as "in one way or another, a lot of people are directly or indirectly involved in and influenced by what goes on with NTP" (Interview 80). Approximately 95% of the scientists working in the National Toxicology Program also have faculty positions at the NIEHS, and the director of the NIEHS is also the director of the NTP. The NTP mandate is to strengthen the science base in toxicology; to develop and validate improved testing methods; and to provide information about potentially toxic chemicals to public health regulatory and research agencies, the scientific and medical communities, and the public (NTP 2002). A significant accomplishment of the NTP has been the development of standardized bioassays for use in toxicology testing and risk assessment:

> We developed protocols for doing dosing, [for] how to interpret results, and *we've succeeded in having those interpretations adopted by both government and industry.* This was a huge challenge. Think of all the factors: gender of animal, strain of animal, feeding cycle, light cycle, care cycle, the number of animals in a cage, the dosing mechanism—whether or not it causes the animal pain or is a feeding method. There are all these things to dispute. But, over time, the American scientific community has bought in to this model of testing science. And during that time, the Institute held the line and maintained funding to develop and validate the models (Interview S27, emphasis added).

Since 1978, the NTP has been responsible also for meeting the Congressional mandate for a list of agents to which a significant number of people in the United States are exposed that are "known" or "reasonably anticipated" to be human carcinogens.[15]

Environmental health scientists at the NIEHS and NTP articulate their work as a form of "public service": "At the NIEHS and NTP, we engage in a special form of public service—producing scientific knowledge that promotes individual and public health."[16] As we have seen, the NIEHS distinguishes itself by emphasizing its public health mission. For example, when asked about the mission of the NTP, a toxicologist elaborated:

> Our studies are used in the regulatory process, but they also relate to the issue of disease prevention, which I think NIH does not do enough on. I think a lot of resources go into treating . . . disease conditions, but if you ask the average person on the street, would they be more interested in a drug to treat a cancer or research to prevent that cancer from having developed? I don't think there's any doubt what the answer will be (Interview S96).

Additionally, many environmental health scientists distinguish their work from "science for the sake of science," arguing that it rather is "largely driven by issues that relate to safety of consumer products, occupational exposures, human exposure from substances in the environment, as well as the effects of chemicals on environmental species" (Schwetz 2001: 3–8). For NTP researchers in particular, this means contributing to "regulatory science" (Jasanoff 1990), that is, research oriented specifically to the needs of the regulatory agencies. However, the line between basic research and regulatory research seems especially porous in the environmental health sciences.[17] Environmental health scientists working in academic research centers, where one might expect to find an orientation to basic research, report that their research agendas also are influenced by the needs of the regulatory agencies:

> The regulatory agendas lead to a need for information. So a large part of environmental health science is driven by what is regulated, what is proposed for regulation, and especially what is set on a regular calendar for re-regulation, like all the Clean Air Act criteria pollutants (Interview S09).

In publications also, NIEHS scientists note that "NIEHS-supported research has also served as the source of information for many of the regulatory standards put forward by the US environmental health regulatory agencies to protect human health" (Olden, Guthrie, & Newton 2001: 1966).

Consequently, in contrast to scientists who draw firm boundaries between their research and its potential political implications, environmental health scientists—and especially those working in toxicology—state rather that "toxicology is a political science" (Interview S42). In making this point, a pathologist described the surprise of researchers who come to the environmental health sciences from other fields and discover that their findings have political consequences:

> Scientists who venture into toxicology sometimes find themselves causing uproars. They're surprised, because they're used to debating cancer pathways in the literature. But, they start one of those debates here and a product is pulled off the shelves (Interview S42).

At the same time, NIEHS administrators engage in extensive boundary work (Gieryn 1999; see also Jasanoff 1990) by emphasizing that the *content* of their science itself must be "apolitical": "integrity and being apolitical . . . is our stock-in-trade . . . anything we deal with is based on the science . . . " (Interview S37). Such comments highlight the charged relationship between environmental health science and environmental regulation.

Regulating Environmental Exposures

> A positive epidemiology or clinical finding really
> is a failure of public health policy.
> Testimony of George Lucier (US GPO 2007: 54)

Beginning in the 1970s, Congress charged a combination of old and new federal agencies with responsibility for assessing the risks of environmental contaminants and formulating regulations to protect the public's health and the health of the environment (Jasanoff 1990). Included in this mandate was the new Environmental Protection Agency (EPA),[18] which was founded in 1970 to "consolidate in one agency a variety of federal research, monitoring, standard-setting and enforcement activities to ensure environmental protection" (Lewis 1985). EPA's mission is to protect human health and to safeguard the natural environment, that is, the air, water, and land, upon which life depends.

The Agency's regulatory authority is constituted in a panoply of laws. Considering the regulation of a single substance—mercury—makes clear the complexity of environmental regulation. The EPA regulates mercury in the environment under the Clear Air Act, the Clean Water Act, the Resource Conservation and Recovery Act, and the Safe Drinking Water Act. Each of these acts provides EPA with the jurisdiction to issues rules and standards governing a different route through which humans may be exposed to mercury. For example, the Clean Air Act includes special provisions for dealing with air toxics emitted from utilities, giving EPA the authority to regulate power plant mercury emissions.[19] Many states also have developed regulations aimed at reducing mercury emissions to air, land, and water; these often are more stringent than those promulgated at the federal level.[20] Additionally, when found in consumer products, mercury is subject to regulatory oversight by other federal agencies. For example, although EPA is charged with assessing and regulating the risks of mercury in fish caught by sport fishers, the FDA is responsible for regulating mercury exposure in commercially caught fish and shellfish.[21] The Consumer Product Safety Commission (CPSC) has regulatory oversight for consumer products, and has issued warnings regarding mercury vapors in herbal remedies sold at botanicas.[22]

At the center of the EPA's efforts to implement its mission is the process of risk assessment, which refers to "the systematic scientific characterization of potential adverse health effects resulting from human exposures to hazardous agents or situations" (NRC 1983: 1). The goal of risk assessment is to determine whether an environmental hazard might cause harm to exposed persons and ecosystems and to inform regulatory decision making.[23] Broadly speaking, risk assessment has four stages: (1) hazard identification—the determination of whether a substance is linked to a particular human health or environmental effect; (2) dose response—the estimation of the relationship between exposure and its potential effects on health; (3) exposure assessment—assessment of the source of pollution, the nature of migration from the source, and the location of people relative to it; and (4) risk characterization—a synthesis of the previous three steps and the uncertainties therein (Corburn 2005: 85–87; see also NRC 1983). Environmental health research has a central role in each stage; however, risk management strategies are shaped also by economic, legal, political, and technological considerations (Faustman & Omenn 1996; NRC 1983). As a toxicologist noted with some frustration, "even when the science is clear," the EPA is required to consult with diverse stakeholders and consider "nonscientific" concerns as part of a complete regulatory review process (Interview P05). Nonetheless, many environmental health scientists are strongly oriented to the goal of informing risk assessment; descriptions of toxicology, in particular, often emphasize its important role in the risk assessment process (Smith 2001). Even more dramatically, a former NTP scientist told me that "the only reason to do toxicology is to address issues in risk assessment" (Interview S81).

Risk assessment and regulation at the EPA generally have focused on the ambient environment, that is, on assessing and controlling, *via public policy*, chemicals in the environment that may pose a threat to human health. There are a few examples of laws in which biological variations among humans are incorporated in regulatory processes. For example, the Clean Air Act of 1990 and the Food Quality Protection Act of 1996 had specific provisions for the protection of sensitive groups within the general population, such as children and people with asthma. Likewise, there are a few instances of regulators recommending that the risks posed by exposure to environmental chemicals be remediated by an individual behavior.[24] However, the predominant approach to protecting the health of the public vis-à-vis environmental risks has been to control the emission and concentration of harmful chemicals in the air, water, and soil.

This population-level approach contrasts with the individual-level approaches, focused rather on clinical interventions and on behavioral and lifestyle factors, that are central to both biomedicine and the "dominant epidemiological paradigm" (Brown 2007). Insofar as health care utilization, behavioral, factors, and lifestyle factors are seen as individual choices, individual-level approaches tend to hold individuals responsible for their health status (Brown 2007: 20; Petersen & Lupton 1996). In contrast, in public policy approaches, the state retains the responsibility that it acquired in the eighteenth or nineteenth century—the precise timing varying across national contexts—to secure the general conditions of public health by maintaining clean air, water, and food (Rose 2001: 6).

These public policy applications of environmental health science, in turn, have reinforced the alignment of environmental health research with public health. The NIEHS and NTP track the uptake of their research by regulatory agencies as a measure of the contribution of their scholarship.[25] Likewise, environmental health scientists emphasize the potential of their research to intervene at the "front end of disease, or disease etiology, and prevention" (US GPO 2007: 21). Among the consequences of the historical alignment of the environmental health sciences with public health and public policy approaches is that, in order to defend their jurisdiction—and maintain their funding—environmental health scientists must articulate their contribution to public health and maintain clear boundaries with biomedicine.

The public policy applications of environmental health science increase the scrutiny given to such science, which is regularly challenged in regulatory reviews and in litigation. In the United States, the centrality of scientific knowledge in environmental regulation and the readiness of the courts to adjudicate complex scientific questions have given litigating parties incentives to reframe fundamentally political and economic cleavages as disputes over scientific evidence (Jasanoff 1995: 67; Michaels 2008).[26] As a toxicologist noted grimly, "The court cases occur when trying to apply [research] findings to regulations" (Interview S38). Such challenges may center on claims about specific, local exposures and their effects on a community's health (Allen 2003; Brown & Mikkelson 1994; Corburn 2005) or on whether and how it is necessary to regulate substances commonly used in industrial manufacturing of widely distributed consumer products (Jasanoff 1995; Markowitz & Rosner 2002).

Both industry and environmental health advocacy groups have established their own research institutes, as well as collaborations with university-based environmental health scientists, as a means of participating more fully in this arena (Brown et al. 2006).[27] Fundamentally, this means that environmental health research is frequently and publicly contested. That said, these contestations take very different forms. As I discuss later in this chapter, environmental health and justice advocates argue broadly for more protective and democratic approaches to environmental risk assessment and regulation. In contrast, in the past half century, regulated industries have

invested significant financial and institutional resources in the politiciza-
tion of scientific uncertainty, seeking to convince the judiciary and the public that the evidentiary base for environmental regulation is "junk science"
(Michaels 2008; Oreskes & Conway 2010; Ong & Glantz 2001).

"Better Living Through Chemistry" [28]

> An improved understanding of environmental
> health risks is important because economic de-
> velopment plays a vital role in the U.S. and world
> economy and to human welfare . . .
> Testimony of Lynn Goldman (US GPO 2007:66)

Today's chemical industry includes companies producing a staggering
array of products that are central to contemporary life. According to the
American Chemistry Council (ACC), the trade group that represents
the $720 billion industry, chemical production in the United States en-
compasses five product segments: pharmaceuticals, basic chemicals (i.e.,
commodity chemicals produced in large volume and with broad applications), specialty chemicals (i.e., low-volume, high-value compounds
with very specific applications), agricultural chemicals (e.g., pesticides
and fertilizers), and consumer products. Our homes are full of chemical products, such as vitamins, prescription and over-the-counter drugs,
vinyl flooring, cosmetics, soaps, lotions, shampoo, pantyhose, DVDs,
diapers, and household cleaners; most of us use multiple chemical substances each day (Altman et al. 2008).

Chemical production has contributed to the expansion of the American
economy and remains a major component of it; the ACC proudly describes
the U.S. economy as "chemistry dependent." Nearly 800,000 people were
directly employed by the chemical industry in 2010, and the ACC estimates that for every job created in the business of chemistry, 5.5 jobs are
created in other sectors of the economy. In 2010, chemical products ac-
counted for 12% of U.S. exports.

Despite the role of chemistry in creating what the ACC calls the
"American standard of living," both the specific *products* of the chemical

industry and the industrial manufacturing *processes* through which they come into being have been the subject of contentious politics for over a century. Concerns about conditions within factories—and their effects on workers' health—gave rise to broader questions about the health consequences of chemical exposures outside these concentrated industrial settings (Seller 1997). For over a hundred years, the chemical industry has contended that its voluntary compliance with health safeguards will be sufficient to protect the health of workers and the public. However, as noted by public health historians, "there have always been those inside and outside of government who believed that voluntary compliance . . . is not sufficient to safeguard the public's health for the reason that industry's financial interests often prevent it from doing what would be socially responsible" (Markowitz & Rosner 2002: 3).

Advocating for Environmental Health and Justice

> To answer the question of why some communities are more affected by some disease, NIEHS must continue to assess the degree to which environmental exposures disproportionately impact specific communities, to understand the effects of multiple and cumulative exposures, and ultimately what types of intervention will effectively reduce those disparities in health burdens.
> Testimony of Peggy Shepard (US GPO 2007: 72)

Another defining characteristic of the environmental health arena is social movement activism focused on issues of environmental health and justice. Since the 1980s, disease-oriented advocacy groups have demanded a voice in decisions about research funding, the inclusion of specific groups in clinical research, and a broader concern for the needs of people who are ill in the process of registering and making available new pharmaceuticals (Epstein 1996, 2007). Environmental health and justice activists share these concerns; however, insofar as they focus on the social structures and processes in and through which people are exposed to environmental hazards (Brown et al. 2003), their scope and critique are broader than those of many health social movement groups. Environmental justice is the principle that "all people and communities are entitled to equal protection of environmental and public health laws and regulations" (Bullard, in Brulle & Pellow 2006). In the United States, the environmental justice movement (EJM) emphasizes particularly the role of racism and poverty in determining exposure to environmental hazards and the irreplaceable role of public policy in redressing injustice (Brulle & Pellow 2006).

Environmental justice emerged as a focus for the NIEHS under the leadership of Dr. Kenneth Olden. In 1994, the NIEHS established extramural funding for the Environmental Justice: Partnerships for Communication Program. The goal of the program is "to enable community residents to more actively participate in the full spectrum of research." Toward this end, the grant application process required three-way partnerships among "a community organization, an environmental health researcher and a health care professional" who committed to work together "to develop models and approaches to building communication, trust and capacity, with the final goal of increasing community participation in the research process."[29] In 1995, the Institute launched the Community-Based Participatory Research (CBPR) Program to promote "active community involvement in the processes that shape research and intervention strategies, as well as in the conduct of research studies." At the center of this program are community-university partnerships focused on environmental health research and interventions.[30] Such collaborations have been complicated by the "inherent disparities in the relationships between a university and the communities that they study"; nonetheless, research conducted under the auspices of this program has contributed to activists' efforts to document health problems in contaminated communities (Cable, Mix, & Hasting 2005: 68–69). In the context of the NIH, "where participatory research is weak to nonexistent," the NIEHS's approach provides a model for successful collaboration between activists and scientists (Brown 2007: 246-248).

In recent years, environmental health activists have become involved in scientific knowledge production, as a part of their advocacy efforts.

For example, they may engage in techniques of *popular epidemiology,* a process in which concerned citizens systematically gather data about environmental health risks and illness in their community (Brown & Mikkelson 1994), or *street science,* the combination of local knowledge with professional scientific expertise (Corburn 2005). Often, these efforts are undertaken as a means of challenging the "dominant epidemiological paradigm" for a disease and demanding new resources for disease prevention or treatment; successful challenges to the dominant epidemiological paradigm are often the result of collaboration between environmental health activists and environmental health scientists (Brown 2007: 37). There are many obstacles to citizen-scientist collaborations, not the least of which is that many environmental activists are committed to the idea that science is not the only legitimate form of expertise in the domain of environmental health and illness (Corburn 2005: 37–40). However, there are an increasing number of examples of collaborations between environmental health activists and sympathetic scientists in formulating hypotheses about the environmental causation of illness in a community (Brown 2007: 37; see also Allen 2003; Sze 2007). Some have suggested that, over time, these collaborations may produce "ruptures" in scientific practices—and institutions—thereby creating opportunities for the transformation of environmental health research (Ottinger & Cohen 2011).[31]

Environmental health and justice activists have also challenged the risk assessment paradigm, suggesting that the precautionary principle would provide better protection (Brown, Mayer, & Linder 2002; Tickner 2003). There are two general versions of the precautionary principle; the strong version states that no action should be taken unless there is full certainty that it will do no harm, and the weak version states that "lack of full certainty is not a justification for preventing an action that might be harmful" (Morris 2000: 1). In regard to environmental regulation, the precautionary principle approach would require that "suspect substances must be held off the market until their potential dangers are more clearly understood and their safety is better established" and would support regulatory action "even before the existing data absolutely prove danger" (Markowitz & Rosner 2002: 6). Proponents of the precautionary principle point out that uncertainties inherent in the scientific risk assessment processes have been used to contest or forestall regulation, such that industrial interests may invest in research specifically intended to "insinuate ambiguity" (Proctor 1995: 102; see also Jasanoff 1990); calls for regulatory delays on the grounds of insufficient and/or incomplete evidence "are a regular part of the PR package of the tobacco, petrochemical, and other industries . . . the net effect is to shift the focus from the need to eliminate a probable hazard to the need to resolve a certain ambiguity" (Proctor 1995: 130). At stake in these debates is the best means of protecting public health.

MECHANISMS OF CHANGE

Collectively, the dynamics among environmental health scientists, regulators, activists, and industry mean that the environmental health sciences fundamentally differ from sciences in which controversy may be concealed within a "core set" of deeply involved researchers (Collins 1985). In contrast, domains of contention, knowledge gaps, and sources of uncertainty within the environmental health sciences are both defined and publicized by the contentious politics of the environmental health arena and its myriad stakeholders.[32] These dynamics have profoundly shaped the foci and pace of research at the NTP and NIEHS: "This [dynamic] is very different than . . . [at] most of the other NIH institutes and extramural constituencies, because they can do their research via the classical scientific approach and don't have this sort of overriding pressure for validation/precision on a short time-frame" (Interview S27). As such, environmental health scientists report that they are strongly motivated to strengthen the certainty and, related, the legitimacy of their research. In contrast to other scientists, environmental health researchers must not only produce knowledge that will meet the standards of their scientific peers, but also ensure that it is robust to both technical and legal challenges by outside parties. Beginning in the 1980s, environmental health scientists began to consider how studying environmental exposures at the molecular genetic level might serve as a means to these interrelated ends.

In some ways, it is unsurprising that environmental health scientists would turn to research on molecular mechanisms of environmental illness as a means of strengthening the certainty and legitimacy of their research. As early as the 1980s, the NTP came under pressure to develop its research on the molecular mechanisms behind responses to environmental chemicals.[33] In 1984, the NTP Board of Scientific Counselor's Ad Hoc Panel on Chemical Carcinogenesis Testing and Evaluation Report recommended that the National Toxicology Program "establish a goal of better understanding mechanisms by developing a battery of short term tests that measures the widest possible number of endpoints (including promotion, transformation, and chemical interaction with oncogenes)" (NTP 1984: 92). Then, again, in 1992, a scientific review panel convened to evaluate the NTP reported that the program "places too much emphasis on testing per se" and not enough on understanding underlying mechanisms through which exposures to specific substances cause adverse outcomes (Stone 1993). "Developing and applying tools of modern toxicology and *molecular biology*" became part of the official mission of the NTP (NTP 2002, 2, emphasis added). As one scientist recalled, there was concern that, unless it found ways to incorporate molecular genetic techniques, "the NTP would be a toxicology program of only historical interest" (Interview S32).

At this time, there was a burgeoning interest in genetics across the life sciences. By the 1990s, molecular genetics and genomics were at the apex of biomedical research in the United States. The power of genetic explanations for human health and illness was manifest in massive public investiture in the Human Genome Project (HGP), as well as in policy debates, popular culture, and a wide variety of research enterprises (Nelkin & Lindee 1994; Lindee 2005). Proponents of the HGP predicted that it would provide a new understanding of "what it means to be a human being" (Bodmer & McKie 1997: vii) and a new sense of our biological possibilities. Simply put, there was a massive genetics bandwagon in the life sciences, replete with new questions, technologies, and training programs, all focused on the molecular vision of life (Fujimura 1996). NIH leaders heralded especially the "revolutionary" implications of molecular genetic and genomic research for clinical practice (Collins 1999).

Environmental health scientists report that the ascendance of molecular genetic research in the life sciences raised concerns about the status of their research, which, on the whole, was not focused at the molecular level. Scientists recalled becoming alarmed by the perception that environmental health research was relatively "not innovative . . . not basic science driven" (Interview S20), especially compared to molecular biology. Such concerns about environmental health science being "behind the leading edge" (Field Notes, NIEHS 2002) had implications for the status and prestige of institutions that fund and implement environmental health research. In articulating his support of initiatives that focus environmental health research at the molecular level, a former director of the NIEHS explained:

> I think we were perceived as not being terribly mainstream and relevant, so we had to change. We had to incorporate modern science, take advantage of new innovations in cell and molecular biology and develop new test systems (Olden, Oral History Interview February 2004).

Or, as molecular epidemiologist put it, by the 1990s, NIEHS was under considerable pressure to establish itself as more than just "a rat toxicology institute" (Field Notes, NIEHS June 2002). Indeed, although even critics aver that "rat toxicology" has made significant contributions to protecting public health and safety, many scientists assign it a lower status than "basic" laboratory research.[34] According to a university-based environmental health scientist, starting in the 1980s, the NIEHS was not "getting as much money as it deserved"; one explanation for this is that it was perceived as "falling behind completely, compared to the rest of NIH" (Interview S20). Some respondents noted also that although the NIEHS has "great stature" by virtue of being part of the NIH, *within* the NIH, the NIEHS has to struggle to overcome being positioned as the "country cousins" (Interview P03) of the Institutes or "NCI [National Cancer Institute] South . . . a copy cat version" (Stone 1993); these are both derogatory references that refer to the NIEHS's North Carolina location to impugn its scientific standing. At the NIEHS, I was told, "The genomics revolution is washing over us. Either we incorporate it or we'll be left behind" (Field Notes, NIEHS July 2002).[35]

At the same time that they rose to the myriad challenges of the genomic revolution, environmental health scientists had to find ways to incorporate genomics into their research in ways that would support their public health mission; as made vivid in their testimonies before Congress in 2007, this constitutes a primary rationale for their jurisdiction and funding. To be sure, environmental health scientists were not alone in seeking to articulate how the genomic revolution could contribute to public health. For example, in 1997, the Centers for Disease Control and Prevention (CDC) opened an Office of Genetics and Disease Prevention (now known as the Office of Public Health Genomics), which was tasked with developing strategies for "assist[ing] public health professionals in promoting health and preventing disease and disability among people for whom the consequences of an inherited risk can be ameliorated."[36] Throughout the late 1990s, the CDC sponsored a series of conference on genetics, public health, and disease prevention.[37] In 2000, an edited volume, entitled *Genetics and Public Health in the 21st Century: Using Genetic Information to Improve Health and Prevent Disease*, presented "a framework for the integration of advances in human genetics into public health practice" (Khoury, Burke, & Thomson 2000). However, the assumption underlying these programs and frameworks was that "genetic information in public health is appropriate in diagnosing, treating and preventing disease, disability, and death among people *who inherit specific genotypes.*"[38] Newborn genetic screening and predisposition testing of individuals from families affected by heritable conditions were oft cited models for how genetics could improve public health (see Khoury, Burke, & Thomson 2000). This individual-level focus on screening and behavior change fit well with the assumption that genomics would allow clinicians to customize interventions to individuals' genotypes.[39] However, it was not well aligned with the public policy and regulatory orientation of the environmental health sciences.

In fact, the challenge of articulating the public health and public policy relevance of developing genomics in the environmental health sciences was accentuated by widespread predictions that the primary contribution of genomics to human health would be a profound personalization of clinical practice. "Personalized medicine"—that is, medical practice in which preventive screening, lifestyle, and dietary modifications, diagnostics, targeted drug therapies and family planning are all tailored to an individual's genetic profile—is the holy grail of contemporary genomics research (e.g., Collins 1999; Feero, Guttmacher, & Collins 2008). Given that individual, clinical biomedical interventions are precisely what environmental health science traditionally is *not*, environmental health researchers were faced with the challenge of how to develop ways of engaging with genomics that strengthened their field, rather than increasing its marginalization.

As we will see, there has been tremendous variation in scientists' strategies for incorporating genomics into environmental health research, risk assessment, and regulation. Starting in the 1980s, and accelerating thereafter, environmental health scientists developed diverse molecular techniques and practices—such as environmental genomics, molecular epidemiology, and toxicogenomics—tailored to the specific questions and struggles at the center of their subfields, as well as the broader challenges posed by the contentious politics of the environmental health arena and the rise of molecular genetics. [40] Although some of these practices built on extant lines of research, others aimed to establish wholly new research foci and techniques. Further, while many of these practices sought to articulate applications of genomics specific to the process of environmental health risk assessment and regulation, others sought to extend the reach of environmental health science into clinical settings, establishing new and potentially lucrative markets for environmental health research. Before turning to those specific practices, however, it is important to examine scientists' broad rationale for the turn to research on gene-environment interaction spanning these fields. The next chapter describes how a "consensus critique" was used to mobilize the struggles and challenges of the environmental health arena in support of the idea that research on gene-environment interaction is essential to the public health mission of the environmental health sciences.

TWO The Consensus Critique

Now that we have a draft of the genome, the next big
challenge is understanding how genes interact with the
environment.

Field Notes, NIH, 2002

As long as the health and the environment . . . environmental
health, is kept as a primary focus, then it [NIEHS] has a
unique role.

Testimony of Stefani Hines (US GPO 2007: 88)

Under what circumstances would environmental health scientists see molecular genetic approaches to understanding human health and illness as an *opportunity,* rather than a threat to the jurisdiction and standing of their field? As one environmental health scientist put it, genetic research—especially as it was being "oversold" as the key to unlocking the mysteries of *all* human health and illness—appeared to many "as much as a barrier as a way to take action" (Interview S50). Following the publication of the first map of the human genome and the revelation that it contains many fewer genes than initially expected, environmental health scientists argued that genomic research had produced the unintended consequence of highlighting the importance of the environment to human health (Olden & White 2005).[1] However, even in advance of this revelation, environmental health scientists had begun to advocate for the idea that gene-environment interaction was critical to understanding human health and illness. Notably, beginning in the mid-1990s, the leadership of the National Institute of Environmental Health Sciences (NIEHS) began promoting a research agenda for the field that focused on gene-environment interaction, broadly defined. To mobilize environmental health scientists to support research on gene-environment interaction, its advocates would have to convince their colleagues that molecular genetic and genomic techniques could advance the public health mission of the environmental health sciences, contribute to efforts to inform public policy, and bolster environmental health research when it is challenged in regulatory reviews and litigation. At the same time, they had to find ways of accommodating the goals and aspirations of environmental health scientists who were eager to establish a "more biomedical" approach to environmental health, which would include individual-level, clinical interventions. Reconciling these multiple and often competing visions of the field was no small feat.

This chapter examines how scientists advocating for research on gene-environment interaction made a case for this new way of thinking about environmental health research. The jumping off place for my analysis is the observation that "the basic problem for skilled social actors is to frame 'stories' that help induce cooperation from people in their group that appeal to their identity, while at the same time using the same stories to frame actions against various opponents" (Fligstein 2001: 113; see also Frickel & Gross 2005).[2] Such identities and narratives may be most powerful when they draw on the extant stock of meanings, beliefs, ideologies, practices, values, rules, and resources already at play in an arena. However, they also have to navigate those same meanings, tensions, and conflicts. For example, the dynamics of contention in the environmental health arena have meant that, to be persuasive, scientists' framing of gene-environment interaction have to appeal to stakeholders with widely divergent, indeed opposed, substantive goals and commitments in the regulatory process.

Scientists advocating for research on gene-environment interaction developed a narrative that included both a diagnosis of the problems and challenges facing the environmental health sciences ("diagnostic framing")[3] and a set of proposed solutions to those problems ("prognostic framing") that highlighted the potential of molecular approaches.[4] As I will demonstrate in the following pages, the social institutions, actors, processes, and especially the politics of the environmental health arena provided "readily available scripts" (Fligstein 2001: 110) for scientists eager to promote research on gene-environment interaction. In particular, scientists mobilized long-standing critiques of the process of environmental health risk assessment and regulation.[5]

At the same time, the dynamics and concerns of the environmental health arena set an important limit on the development of narratives about gene-environment interaction and its potential contributions. That is, while identifying problems and solutions to the challenges of environmental health research, risk assessment, and regulation, advocates of research on gene-environment interaction have exercised care not to wholly undermine the legitimacy of the current risk assessment paradigm. This is not only because the current system serves as the basis for environmental health regulation, and thus public health protection, nor simply because the regulatory agencies themselves are key stakeholders in this process. Rather, as described in Chapter 5, it is because the current system provides the standards by which new, molecular risk assessment techniques are evaluated. As such, framing processes must answer the question, "If this works, why fix it?" without portraying the current system as so "broke" as to be illegitimate (Interview S41).

I call the narrative scientists crafted in response to these manifold challenges a *consensus critique*. A consensus critique represents an effort to bring stakeholders together around a set of shared concerns that transcend their substantive political, economic, and/or social differences. It diagnoses problems and proposes solutions in ways that are acceptable to actors who seek divergent—and often opposed—ends. Often, this is accomplished by focusing on potential improvements to a central social *process*, while remaining agnostic about how such improvements may change outcomes, such as the balance of power or opportunities for success among stakeholders. Related, a consensus critique might orient to core values—such as truth or fairness—that are nearly impossible for stakeholders to disavow (though, they may contest their meaning). As such, consensus critiques facilitate collective action in politically contentious arenas.

However, even as it brings stakeholders together around set of shared concerns, a consensus critique will sideline or obfuscate issues that lie beyond its specific definition of core problems and proposed solutions. Social actors whose concerns are excluded by a consensus critique will have good cause, then, to challenge the agenda set in response to it. Consequently, the collective action facilitated by a consensus critique may give rise to the next loci of contention in an arena.

In advocacy for molecular approaches to environmental health research, the consensus critique has centered on technical challenges inherent to the current risk assessment process that a wide variety of stakeholders perceive as salient concerns. It has three main emphases. First, it highlights the challenges inherent in extrapolating from laboratory-based toxicological research— often conducted using highly standardized animal models exposed to high doses of one chemical over a short period of time—to complex interactions between human bodies and their environments in everyday settings. Second, it points to the fact that many more chemicals are in use than have been evaluated in risk assessment by the federal regulatory agencies. Third, it calls attention to questions about how to assess the risks that a substance poses to individuals who are at the sensitive end of the toxic response continuum. The success of this narrative hinges, in large part, on the fact that, although scientists, regulators, industry, and health advocates tend to disagree vehemently about the *outcomes* of particular risk assessments, they tend to agree nonetheless that the *process* itself could be improved. The consensus critique, in its firm faith in the promise of the further scientization of environmental health governance via molecular genetics, thus provides a rationale for research on gene-environment interaction, while eliding the substantive political and economic interests underlying conflict in the environmental health arena.

In addition to obviating the substantive differences of stakeholders in favor of a technical critique of risk assessment, the consensus critique offers scientists a remarkable and consequential degree of interpretive flexibility. While positioning research on gene-environment interaction as the solution to "intractable problems" (Olden 2002: 275), it never defines exactly what gene-environment interaction is, how one should study it, or which molecular genetic technologies or applications thereof offer the greatest promise. As such, it has allowed environmental health scientists to develop research agendas focused on widely varied definitions of gene-environment interaction. Similarly, the consensus critique has opened up space for epidemiologists, toxicologists, and other researchers to develop their own subfield-specific responses to it.

This flexibility, however, has limits. Specifically, the consensus critique fails to account for the social structural issues—such as racial segregation and poverty—that shape disparities in environmental exposures in the United States. Few environmental health scientists call attention to this omission. However, as shown in Chapter 6, the limits of scientization feature prominently in EJ activists' concerns about the ascendance of gene-environment interaction in the environmental health sciences. As such, the consensus critique is an important starting point for understanding not only how research on gene-environment interaction has emerged in the environmental health sciences, but with what biopolitical consequences.

THE CONSENSUS CRITIQUE

"The Intractable Problems"

The diagnostic component of the consensus critique centers on the limitations of the current risk assessment process. NIEHS administrators characterize these limitations as "the intractable problems" that "have long characterized the field"; they include questions about the ability of extant techniques to assess "intrinsic toxicity to humans, variation in susceptibility, crosstalk or interaction between agents in mixtures, and the type, pattern and magnitude of human exposure to chemicals" (Olden 2002: 275). Toxicologists highlight especially the challenges inherent to the two-year rodent cancer bioassay, which is the current gold standard for carcinogenicity testing:

> There are major obstacles in toxicology and this has been obvious to a lot of people: extrapolation from animals to humans, all the issues about

exposure, because with the rats, you're giving a large dose over a concentrated period of time but humans are exposed to varying doses over
longer periods of time and exposed to mixtures . . . and then there are
issues of nutrition and genetic susceptibility (Interview S32, emphasis
added).

In addition to identifying the challenges of toxicology testing, the consensus critique emphasizes the *uncertainty* that derives from issues surrounding the extrapolation of data derived from *in vivo* testing in animal
model systems to establish the risks to humans. This aspect of the consensus critique is highlighted especially by regulatory scientists. For
example, one regulator stated starkly, "people . . . worry about the relevance of animal studies" (Interview P03). Another regulatory scientist
expressed a similar concern by stating that the two-year rodent bioassay
"gives you the answers: (1) this does cause cancer in rodents; (2) this
does not cause cancer in rodents; (3) this might cause cancer in rodents.
Then, you have to extrapolate to humans. This entire process is difficult,
slow, and expensive" (Interview P02).

Second, and related, environmental health scientists emphasize the
consequences of expensive and time-consuming nature of the two-year
rodent cancer bioassays, specifically, the tremendous number of high production chemicals that have not yet been tested. In fact, scholars estimate
that of the chemicals on the EPA's high production volume list (that is,
chemicals produced in high volume in industry), an estimated 93% lack
basic chemical screening tests, and 43% have not been subject to basic
toxicology testing (Brown, Mayer, & Linder 2002; see also Altman et al.
2008). In explaining her enthusiasm for genomics research, a toxicologist
referred to the need to "break the bottleneck" in testing and "deal with
the backlog of chemicals that are still waiting to be tested" (Field Notes
August 2002). Another toxicologist stated:

> The idea is that we'd like to be doing it better. We'd like to be doing
> it cheaper. We'd like to be doing it more quickly. Because you know,
> at eight compounds a year, and millions and millions of dollars
> [per compound] we're never even going to make a dent in every-
> thing that's out there that probably needs to be tested (Field Notes
> August 2002).

In reflecting on his years as director of the NIEHS and National
Toxicology Program (NTP), Olden also invoked issues of efficiency in
reference to his support of efforts to establish new, molecular techniques
for use in risk assessment:

> We were just using a few very standard assays that had been in existence
> for years, and there are still people who tell me we should still be doing
> that. But I felt that we were not providing a very good product—a qual-
> ity product; and the efficiency was very poor. In other words, we were
> spending too much money and generating very little useful information
> (Olden, Oral History Interview July 2004).

Even scientists who believe that animal bioassays provide the most reliable data for risk assessment note that the current system is unable to keep
pace with the demand for testing. In fact, concerns about the backlog of
chemicals awaiting assessment dates back to the NCI's Cancer Bioassay
Program, the precursor of the NTP (Smith 1979). However, the volume of
testing has decreased over time, as the studies conducted have become
more complex and costly. As this toxicologist noted, "One change that
has occurred over the years is a decrease, a significant decrease in the
number of chemicals that NTP studies for carcinogenicity. Whereas in
the early '80s there were about 50 per year, in the '90s it drifted down to
somewhere around 10 per year" (Interview S96).

Third, the consensus critique positions unexamined variation in
susceptibility among humans as a source of uncertainty in the risk assessment process:

> We do most of our assessments based upon the typical American. We
> think there is going to be so many cancers averted, so many reproduc-
> tion problems and so on and so forth. We do not consider the fact that
> individuals are different . . . granted, we do look at subpopulations . . .
> but [not] . . . from a genomic point of view, whereas, in fact, that's really
> what we're talking about (Interview P03).

Currently, risk assessors take the value that toxicology testing has determined to be an acceptable exposure limit for a standard human (e.g.,
the no observed effect level [NOEL]) and multiply it by ten (Smith 1996).
Although many regulatory scientists believe that this is a conservative

practice that is successful in protecting susceptible individuals, such ten-fold factors are seen as arbitrary and burdensome by regulated industries (Interview P03), and environmental health advocates question whether they are truly protective (Interview P06). This also raises the more general issue of how to protect particularly vulnerable individuals, who, with few exceptions, are not specifically protected under existing laws and regulations.

In their articulations of the consensus critique, environmental health scientists highlight the fact that such broad domains of uncertainty provide opportunities for expensive and time-consuming legal challenges to risk assessments (Michaels 2008). In the words of a toxicologist, "people who want to promote political uncertainty will use scientific uncertainty as a basis" (Field Notes, NIEHS July 2002).[6] However, even as they acknowledge the political (and, arguably, economic) interests that motivate controversy in the environmental health arena, scientists emphasize the potential of molecular genetic and genomic techniques to address the uncertainties and limitations in current toxicological testing practices and to improve the capacity of environmental health research to contribute to risk assessment and regulation (e.g., Paules et al. 1999; Olden 2002; Simmons & Portier 2002).

The Prognostic Promise of Molecular Techniques

The prognostic component of the consensus critique positions gene-environment interaction, broadly construed, as a means of addressing these challenges. Advocates of molecular genetic and genomic approaches claim that by reducing the scientific uncertainty that has previously made environmental health research particularly vulnerable to challenges in the context of risk assessment and regulation, it will be possible to definitively and more rapidly assess a larger volume of chemicals. In general, the molecular genetic and genomic technologies and methods championed by advocates of this approach vary substantially depending on their subfields.

Toxicologists have been particularly concerned to articulate how genomic technologies can reshape toxicology testing. For example, they point to four distinct, though not mutually exclusive, means by which gene expression profiling, the signal technology of toxicogenomics, could reduce uncertainty in the risk assessment process. First, they promote gene expression profiles as a means of elucidating mechanisms of toxicity and enhancing the knowledge base of toxicology. Second, they suggest that gene expression profiles may provide a basis for a new, molecular rationale for the classification (and reclassification) of toxicants (that is, grouping toxicants that share similar gene expression profiles). Third, and related, scientists are actively pursuing the potential of gene expression profiles to enable the *prediction* of the toxicity of unknown compounds and thereby provide a basis for their classification (that is, without undergoing the two-year rodent bioassay). Fourth, they point to the possibility that gene expression profiles could serve as new molecular biomarkers of genetic susceptibility. Together, scientists argue, these innovations could increase the speed, efficiency, predictive capacity, and specificity of toxicology testing, making risk assessment more comprehensive and more certain (Bartosiewicz et al. 2000; Bartosiewicz et al. 2001; Burchiel et al. 2001; Fielden & Zacharewski 2001; Hamadeh et al. 2002a; Hamadeh et al. 2002b; Paules et al. 1999; Pennie et al. 2000; Tennant 2001).

Some foci of the consensus critique have been taken up differently across specific subfields. The issue of human genetic variation in response to environmental exposures is the most prominent example of this; it is a central focus of initiatives in epidemiology and toxicology, as well as being the defining focus of the emerging field of environmental genomics. In the context of risk assessment, research on genetic susceptibility to environmental exposures is promoted as a means of providing more precise estimations of risk for *specific* humans and subpopulations thereof, replacing a one-size-fits-all approach with one that acknowledges variation among human bodies. Testifying in support of the NIEHS Institute's Budget for 2002, then NIEHS Director Olden told the U.S. Congress that "individuals can vary by more than *two-thousand fold* in their capacity to repair or prevent damage following exposure to toxic agents in the environment" (Olden, Fiscal Year 2002 Budget Statement, emphasis added). This argument has been prominent also in publications by the NIEHS leadership:

> At present, human genetic variation is not implicitly considered in estimating dose-response relationships, nor is it considered when

setting exposure limits. Data on the prevalence and characteristics of susceptibility genes offers the potential to reduce the guesswork in risk assessment and therefore it is likely that the ability to issue fair and appropriate regulations concerning human hazards will increase markedly (Olden & Wilson 2000).

As this statement makes clear, the argument can be "extended" (Snow et al. 1986) to speak to "both sides" of regulatory battles; even though they may disagree about what "fair and appropriate regulation" would look like, industry, activists, and regulators cannot help but agree that it is a worthy goal.

At the same time, the problem of human genetic variation in response to environmental exposures is a focus of research in environmental genomics and molecular epidemiology that seeks to develop new *clinical* tools for identifying persons at risk, in addition to providing surveillance, early intervention, or prophylaxis to prevent disease onset. As I detail in the following chapter, NIEHS administrators frame research on genetic susceptibility as an effort to be "responsive to the needs of the American people" (Interview 27), particularly people's need to understand "Why me?" in the context of illness: "my friend smoked the same number of cigarettes, we worked in the same industry, and why do I [have cancer]?" (Interview S37). The flexibility of the consensus critique is part of its appeal to a wide variety of stakeholders.

Negotiating Limits

In contrast to the domains of contentious politics, where such narratives are more frequently put to work to mobilize collective action, environmental health scientists who advocate for molecular genetic and genomic research face a unique challenge. Specifically, they have to make a case for a transforming the practices of environmental health science, without thoroughly undermining extant processes of environmental health research, risk assessment, and regulation. This system remains a critical part of the public health infrastructure and, as shown in Chapter 5, it also is integral to their efforts to validate new, molecular techniques. This challenge also has shaped the particular form and foci of the consensus critique.

Scientists use three primary strategies in seeking to promote molecular genetic and genomic techniques for use in testing and risk assessment without delegitimizing current practices and the regulatory policies that rely on them. First, many statements in favor of new techniques emphasize the new *molecular* levels of analysis made possible by molecular genetics and genomic techniques, with the goal of "moving beyond classical toxicology" (NCT 2002). The argument here is that, although current toxicology and risk assessment provide the best possible system at what environmental health scientists call the "phenomenological level," genomics offers an innovative means of conducting toxicological research "down at the molecular level" (Field Notes, NIEHS July 2002). One hoped-for consequence of molecular-level research is that it will illuminate the pathways through which chemicals perturb biological functioning and create toxic effects, as, in the words of a regulatory scientist, "oft times . . . we have no idea in the world how some effect comes about" (Interview P02).[7] Thus, scientists claim that that the effects observed at the phenomenological level are real, albeit poorly understood. Similarly, a molecular epidemiologist argued, "Toxicology needs to go beyond kill 'em and count 'em" (Interview S26). This framing of extant practices as both effective and limited is evident also in a paper about toxicogenomics in *Science*, which described toxicology as both "an imprecise science" and "a time honored way of identifying human health risks" (Lovett 2000: 536).

Second, advocates of molecular genetic and genomic techniques argue that they will provide a means of doing toxicological risk assessment that is quicker and less expensive and that satisfies the demands of the animal rights movement for reductions in animal testing. This comment implies that, although current testing regimens provide accurate data, they are inadequate for testing "everything that's out there" (Interview S27). For example, scientists suggest that genomic techniques could be used to set priorities for toxicology testing at the NTP, thereby increasing its efficacy, given limitations in available time and money for testing:

> The Program has always been interested in looking at alternative methods, other short-term tests that might provide indications of risk. These are extremely valuable in screening and prioritizing chemicals. So, for

example, if you had 50 chemicals and you could only study 10, which ones would you choose? (Interview S96).

Framing the potential contribution of new techniques in this way emphasizes the fiscal and social costs of contemporary toxicological techniques, while leaving their scientific validity unscathed.

Thirdly, scientists emphasize the possibility that molecular genetic and genomic techniques will expand the range of applications of environmental health research. For example, while acknowledging the traditional relationship between environmental health science and environmental regulation, some environmental health scientists frame gene-environment interaction as a means of also developing a range of behavioral and clinical interventions that could improve public health. Advocacy for "a more biomedical environmental health" (Interview S20), which integrates "lifestyle prescriptions" to minimize the risks of exposure or new pharmaceutical interventions to prevent harmful consequences of exposure (Olden, Guthrie, & Newton 2001), does not impugn the current regulatory regime. Rather, it points to a different approach entirely.

Only rarely, and always "off the record," would an environmental health scientist offer an unequivocal critique of risk assessment. For example, this scientist stated: "Risk assessment to me is a black box nightmare. They're making very important decisions based on very limited information. They have a legal obligation to make decisions. But the data is just terrible. So, there is real temptation to use new approaches, because anything is better than nothing, which is what they have now" (Field Notes 2002). Another scientist commented: "Risk assessment is where magic happens, and you have to be careful when you go there . . . . The fact that somebody does some science doesn't make risk assessment less magic" (Field Notes 2001).

More often, using limited frames, proponents of molecular genetics and genomics have been able to promote molecular genetic and genomic technologies as a means of improving toxicology and risk assessment, without discrediting current techniques and standards. This has been critical both to maintaining the legitimacy of the NIEHS, the NTP, and the regulatory system that their research supports and, related, to bringing to the table a wide variety of stakeholders in risk assessment and regulation.

THE MULTIPLE MEANINGS OF GENE-ENVIRONMENT INTERACTION

The interpretive flexibility of the consensus critique has also played an important role in these processes. The consensus critique states that there are limitations to current methods within the environmental health sciences and proposes that molecular genetic techniques offer a way of improving the reliability and validity of environmental health research. However, it never specifies techniques, nor does it offer a precise operational definition of gene-environment interaction. Because gene-environment interaction therefore can encompass a wide range of research foci and techniques, its advocates have been able to garner the support of scientists with disparate research agendas and commitments.

Gene-environment interaction has multiple meanings, which have been shaped by the specific organizational contexts and intellectual lineages of environmental health scientists.[8] To begin, some scientists define gene-environment interaction as the study of the inherited individual and subpopulation genetic susceptibilities that make some people more vulnerable than others to being harmed by environmental exposures. For example, speaking at a meeting of environmental health and justice activists in New York City in 2002, Samuel Wilson, then the Deputy Director of the NIEHS, explained:

> Genes controlling responses to environmental factors have variations in their DNA sequences. That's just a fact that we've begun to appreciate. We see that there are variations. There are many examples where a combination of an exposure and a gene variant are required for an adverse health effect. This is the gene-environment interaction concept (Field Notes 2002).

The identification of individuals and subpopulations that are genetically susceptible to the effects of environmental exposures is a relatively new goal for the environmental health sciences. Toxicologists often explained this new focus to me in terms of their increasing interest in the two outlier populations on a dose-response curve, depicted in Figure 1[9]:

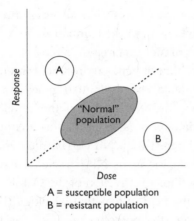

A = susceptible population
B = resistant population

Figure 1.   Dose-response curve.

Previously, susceptible populations and resistant populations were identified primarily so that they could be excluded from analysis (i.e., to avoid misestimating the effects on the "normal" population) (Hattis 1996). However, as detailed in the following chapter, environmental health scientists interested in human genetic variation in response to environmental chemicals define susceptibility (and, less often, resistance) as a primary focus of their research.

In a second definition of gene-environment interaction, environmental health scientists contend that in order to understand—and intervene in—the effects of environmental exposures on human health, one must identify their effects on genes and gene expression. For example, a molecular epidemiologist explained that her research on gene-environment interaction focused on:

> . . . actually proving that people had these compounds, these carcinogenic compounds, inside them . . . [and] had damaged DNA because of these carcinogens. See, before that, all we had was the industrial hygiene people [who] would tell us, "yes, these people have inhaled carcinogens or PAHs, or benzene or something." And maybe there were some assays, some urine-type assays, showing that people were excreting them. But the molecular [biomarkers], the adduct assays were the first to show that *these compounds actually interacted with, and permanently bound to things like DNA* (Interview S12, emphasis added).

This definition encompasses research on environmental mutagenesis, DNA repair mechanisms (and their impairment), and epigenetics; it is also a defining focus of molecular epidemiology.

This second definition of gene-environment interaction—with its focus on how environmental chemicals affect genes and their functioning—was already built into the infrastructure of the NIEHS and NTP. From its inception, genetic damage was "identified as a component of environmental hazards" of interest at the NIEHS (Barrett, Oral History Interview February 2004). During the 1970s, NIEHS scientists (many of whom had transferred from the Biology Division of the Oak Ridge National Laboratory) established the field of genetic toxicology (Frickel 2004), which focused originally on "the potential of chemicals to induce heritable changes in germ cells that lead to genetic disorders in subsequent generations" (Shelby, Oral History Interview April 2004).[10] Many of these researchers shared an interest in developing short-term tests to "study the mechanisms of chemically induced DNA damage and to assess the potential genetic hazard of chemicals to humans" (Tennant et al. 1987). In the early 1970s, the work of Bruce Ames and his colleagues made a strong connection between DNA damage and cancer and provided a relatively easy mutagenesis bioassay—the *Salmonella* test—to identify carcinogens (Ames et al. 1973).[11] Soon thereafter, following the advocacy of prominent environmental health scientists, short-term tests for mutagenesis were "enshrined in regulatory requirements and in biomedical research more generally as carcinogenicity screens" (Frickel 2004). As such, there was significant genetic toxicological infrastructure and expertise at the NIEHS and NTP.

Research on the molecular mechanisms of carcinogenesis has been another site for the development of research on gene-environment interaction at NIEHS. As Carl Barrett, formerly the Scientific Director of NIEHS, recalled, "There was not much of an emphasis in the early days, the first decade of the NIEHS, on cancer because there was a cancer institute. So there was . . . an intentional focus away from cancer to distinguish NIEHS from NCI [National Cancer Institute]." However, beginning in the late 1970s, "there was a growing interest and involvement in cancer [research] within the institute" (Barrett, Oral History Interview

February 2004). In 1987, the NIEHS founded the Laboratory of Molecular Carcinogenesis (LMC) and charged it to "elucidate the genes involved in the [cancer] process and use that information to understand how the environment impacts it" (Barrett, Oral History Interview February 2004). By focusing on the role of environmental chemicals in cancer causation, the LMC added complexity to then ascendant scientific explanations of genes as the primary basis of cancer causation (Fujimura 1996): "While we were doing the molecular analysis, we were also studying how a number of environmental chemicals worked . . . [and] we developed a paradigm for thinking about how environmental health worked—that health and disease [are] a consequence of the interaction between ones genes and environment over time" (Barrett, Oral History Interview February 2004).

In addition to the flexibility of this paradigm across varied scientific disciplines (with their different definitions of gene-environment interaction and ways of studying it) and stakeholders in the environmental health arena (with their different investments in the process of risk assessment and regulation), it has been importantly flexible *over time*.

[All the major genomics initiatives at NIEHS] were part of a greater strategy of trying to bring new technologies and new concepts to bear in terms of environmental health sciences, and they really are *extensions of the concept of gene-environment over time* (Barrett, Oral History Interview February 2004).

The ability of the concept of gene-environment interaction to be extended over time has meant, in practice, that new technologies and research agendas can be subsumed under its aegis. For example, in 1997, the major genomics initiative at NIEHS centered on sequencing genes that conferred susceptibility to environmental exposures (i.e., environmental genomics); by 2001, NIEHS had also launched a major effort to use microarrays to study the effects of environmental chemicals on gene expression (i.e., toxicogenomics). More recently, researchers have promoted the promise of epigenetics by referring to gene-environment interaction (Olden et al. 2011). Research on gene-environment interaction has been undertaken with a staggering array of techniques, including high-throughput gene sequencers, molecular biomarkers, cDNA and protein microarrays, genome-wide association studies, and quantitative PCR, to name just a few. Thus, the concept of gene-environment interaction has engaged environmental health scientists even as the substantive foci, technologies, and concepts at the center of research shift and change.

CRITIQUING THE CONSENSUS CRITIQUE

Despite its rhetorical strengths and successes, not all environmental health scientists have been persuaded by the consensus critique. NIEHS administrators freely admitted that scientists whom they referred to as "traditional toxicologists" were "not happy" with changes underway at the NIEHS and NTP and referred me to their colleagues for "dissenting" opinions (Field Notes, NIEHS 2002).

However, given the scope of the proposed and ongoing changes to their field, it was surprisingly difficult to find scientists who were critical of research on gene-environment interaction or, related, the development of molecular genetic and genomic techniques for risk assessment. In the one overt exception, a scientist referred to toxicogenomics as "crapola" and contested the relevance of research on molecular mechanisms to the NTP's public health mission:

> . . . everybody coming out of school in the last 15 years are all molecular, DNA is the answer, which [it] may be and which is fine. But [at NTP] we need some people with practicality. We need some people with [skills in] toxicology . . . empirical descriptive toxicology. [If] you find out something causes cancer, then let somebody else mess around with the mechanism. . . . I don't want to know how it does it . . . I want to know, "Is this safe?" (Interview S97).

Further, a few scientists took issue with the promise of individual techniques of studying gene-environment interaction, noting, for example their "skepticism" regarding research being done in specific transgenic mouse models (even while endorsing research being done with other transgenic mouse models) (Interview S96). However, on the whole, those scientists identified by their peers as dissenters commented on the successes of their field, built on traditional approaches to assessing risks and preventing exposures, rather than offering a critique of emerging molecular approaches to environmental health research. For example, a toxicologist—who in the course of our interview told a colleague who dropped by that I was there to talk with her as "one of those who isn't in the 'genes will save us' camp"—commented: "My interest is in, what can we change to make people healthier? We can change exposures. . . . You can't change your gene pool" (Interview S28).

As with the consensus critique, the counternarratives offered by dissenting scientists were based on key aspects of the field's identity, including its relationship to public health and its unique contributions to regulatory decision making and public policy. For example, when I asked a toxicologist about his perspective on the potential of molecular genetic techniques to improve toxicology testing and risk assessment, he responded by highlighting the successes of the NTP in preventing environmentally associated diseases:

> I think the NTP does probably more than any other program on issues related to disease prevention. . . . How many lives were saved by reducing human exposure? That's hard to determine with accuracy. But we know that there are carcinogenic agents in our environment and workplace, risks are elevated, and it is our goal to provide scientific information that can be used to reduce human risk from environmental agents. . . . That is, as far as I'm concerned, the major mission of NTP . . . Our role is to provide the science so that decisions are made that are protective of public health (Interview S96).

Similarly, a scientist contended that the rodent cancer bioassay program—despite its limitations—has succeeded in providing "EPA with the ammunition that they may need." (Field notes, NIEHS June 2002). Even scientists who, on the whole, supported the adoption of molecular genetic and genomic techniques pointed to the historic successes of current methods of toxicology testing. For example, a molecular epidemiologist acknowledged that "The other side . . . is that this way has served the public well. If you screen out the things that kill rats, you will protect a lot of people" (Interview S26). A toxicologist pointed out that repeated efforts to replace animal bioassays have come to naught: " . . . other thoughtful people have attempted to replace the bioassay with something, as we say—faster, more accurate, cheaper and less animals—and that's our goal. But in the 25 years I've been in this [field] there's been a thousand substitutes, none of which have worked" (Interview S97).

More rarely, scientists would suggest that by absorbing scarce resources and introducing new forms of uncertainty into toxicology testing, new molecular techniques would impede and delay the regulatory process. In part, this concern is about the distribution of resources within the environmental health sciences and the possibility that investing in new techniques will divert support from current toxicity testing programs:

> . . . people who want the environment protected are concerned that, by siphoning resources away from the chronic studies that are already readily accepted by the agencies, into something that may not be as accepted by them, is to make either a longer time to regulatory intervention, or preclude it, actually preclude it (Interview S41).

Even more to the point, a university-based environmental health researcher commented: "when NIEHS spends so much of their money on the genetic revolution, I wonder how much of that they can really devote to . . . more environmental issues" (Interview S50).

A related set of issues centers on the possibility that the chemical industry could use the uncertainties attendant to new molecular approaches as a rationale for delaying regulatory review of their products. In fact, some scientists suggested that the chemical industry's interest in genomic approaches to risk assessment was motivated precisely by the potential of new and complex techniques to complicate and delay regulatory processes:

> [They] see it as a tool, a delaying action . . . [They say] "I'm going to do this study first to guide me and it will take me two years." And the regulatory agency says, "okay go ahead." So, that means two more years that industry can use the product without any regulatory [oversight] . . . it's a great delaying tactic. Any new technology, it's always a good delaying tactic for environmental health risk assessments (Interview S41).

Officially, the chemical industry favors the development of new "-omics" technologies that can be used in risk assessment (Henry et al.

2002). However, scientists disagree as to whether, to what extent, and for what reasons, the chemical industry supports the development of genomic techniques. Although some scientists claimed that industry supports these technologies for their ability to delay regulatory reviews, others suggested that "Officially, they're very supportive, but really they're not interested at all . . . in the development of better ways of finding out that their products are toxic" (Field Notes, NIEHS 2002). Others noted that establishing a consensus about the applications of new technologies was likely to require significant effort,[12] because even having "more . . . confidence in the models that you use . . . doesn't mean they won't still be controversial and there won't be the arguments from industry and public interest groups, what's safe and what isn't" (Interview S81). Such comments were the only overt acknowledgement that the various parties interested in the development of molecular genetic research and technologies in the environmental health sciences hold very different substantive goals vis-à-vis risk assessment.

In fact, the broader politics of environmental health and especially environmental justice remain almost completely absent from the consensus critique and appear only rarely in the counternarratives of dissenting scientists. Neither diagnostic nor prognostic framing of research on gene-environment interaction tends to draw on the issues of racism and environmental justice raised by environmental justice activists.[13] In their talks to meetings of activists and, more rarely in publications, environmental health scientists claim that research on gene-environment interaction will help us to understand and ameliorate health disparities in the U.S. (e.g., Olden and White 2005). However, many of the solutions proposed in such articles center not on remediating environmental injustices, but rather on identifying genetically susceptible populations[14] and using genomics to better target pharmaceuticals according to "race specific drug response" (Olden and White 2005).

On the rare occasion that scientists raised issues of inequity, it was most often as a counternarrative vis-à-vis the consensus critique. For example, a scientist renowned for his research on lead poisoning in children—a condition marked by dramatic disparities by socioeconomic status (SES) and racial background—commented:

> It's just that to the extent that we think we can understand the genetic contributions to different diseases and solve the world's problems without addressing environmental pollutants or inequity in our systems, I think we're really fooling ourselves . . . I think *scientists have to confront poverty just as much as they confront genetics* (Interview S50, emphasis added).

As we will see in Chapter 6, the omission from the consensus critique of broader social factors, such as poverty and racism, associated with environmental exposure and its focus rather on technical aspects of research and risk assessment have shaped the responses of environmental health and justice activists to research on gene-environment interaction.

FROM PROGNOSTICS TO PRACTICE

The dynamics of contention in the arena of environmental health shape the practices and meanings of environmental health science in the United States. In particular, the dynamics of contention surrounding risk assessment provide readily available scripts for scientists advocating for research focused on gene-environment interaction. These scientists frame the limitations and uncertainties inherent to toxicology testing, in general, and the two-year rodent cancer bioassay, in particular, as the "intractable problems" that undermine their science, jeopardize the standing of their research and institutions, and impede their ability to contribute fully to public health efforts. The consensus critique, then, points to the possibility that, by addressing the technical challenges of toxicology testing, risk assessment, and regulation, molecular genetics and genomics will solve the ongoing dilemmas of environmental health research and governance. As I detail in Chapter 5, the consensus critique has been taken up by myriad stakeholders in the environmental health arena, including, importantly, the regulatory agencies.

The broad appeal of the consensus critique hinges on three of its major characteristics. First, in focusing only on the technical limitations of toxicology testing and risk assessment, the consensus critique elides the substantive political and economic stakes that drive conflict in the environmental health arena. By offering a "story of control" (Stone 2001) that contends that "a tolerated but unwanted state of affairs can now be alleviated through newly available courses of action" (Keller 2009: 49), the consensus critique appeals to stakeholders who actually hope for very different—and, indeed, opposing— substantive outcomes from regulatory reviews. Second, while criticizing extant methods of toxicology testing and risk assessment, the consensus critique stops short of undermining the legitimacy of extant methods and the institutions that rely on them. Third, while positioning research on gene-environment interaction and the application of molecular techniques in risk assessment as a solution to the challenges facing the environmental health sciences, the consensus critique never specifically defines gene-environment interaction, nor does it champion particular technologies. As such, the consensus critique offers environmental health scientists substantial flexibility in developing new research agendas and practices. It has served as a rationale for developing diverse forms of environmental health research, including environmental genomics, molecular epidemiology, toxicogenomics and, more recently, epigenetics.

The relative absence of resistance to the consensus critique is quite remarkable. With only very rare exceptions, even scientists identified by their peers as critical of molecular genetics and genomics in the environmental health sciences did not overtly challenge its tenets. Those who did express concerns tended to focus on problems with specific molecular techniques. A few more noted the possibility that genomics initiatives could have the unfortunate unintended consequences of introducing new uncertainties, consuming scarce resources, and thereby delaying the regulation of potential environmental hazards. Some scientists suggested that there is resistance to "-omics" within the chemical industry, despite its official endorsement of their development for use in risk assessment. However, as elaborated in Chapter 6, EJ activists have been among the only stakeholders in the environmental health arena to directly challenge the assumptions of the consensus critique; they criticize especially its complete lack of attention to the social, economic, and political dynamics that make communities of color especially vulnerable to environmental exposures.

The consensus critique makes a broad case for research on gene-environment interaction and the development of molecular genetic and genomic techniques as a means of improving risk assessment and regulation. As environmental health scientists have shifted their research foci to gene-environment interaction and to the molecular level, what this actually means for their daily practices has varied tremendously. In large part, this is because research on gene-environment interaction has been profoundly shaped by the traditions, challenges, and dispositions of different approaches *within* the environmental health sciences. The next two chapters examine how scientists have assembled particular sets of molecular research practices—environmental genomics and molecular epidemiology—and how the body, the environment, and its interactions are defined, measured, and acted on in each.

THREE Susceptible Bodies

These studies challenge a fundamental tenet of toxicology
dating back to the 17th century; that is, that the dose makes
the poison. We now know that it is the host, plus the dose
and the time of exposure, that makes the poison.

Dr. Kenneth Olden, Director, NIEHS

Fiscal Year 2001 Budget Request[1]

In the late twentieth century, the idea that all human disease is a genetic phenomenon became embedded in the practices and policies of biomedicine, popular understanding of bodies, and beliefs about health and
illness. The rising power of genetic explanations, fueled by increasing
investments in genetic research, was perceived by many environmental
health scientists as a significant challenge to their field, especially given
its jurisdictional focus on the role of the environment in shaping human health and illness. As described in Chapter 1, many environmental

An earlier version of the history presented in this chapter appears in Shostak, S., P. Conrad,
and A.V. Horwitz. "Sequencing and Its Consequences: Path Dependence and the Relationships Between Genetics and Medicalization." *American Journal of Sociology* 114(S1):
S287–S316. Copyright © 2008 University of Chicago Press.

health scientists expressed concern that new, molecular approaches to studying and understanding human health and illness threatened to make their research and their institutions obsolete; "the whole world is genes now," commented a toxicologist (Interview S28). At the National Institute of Environmental Health Sciences (NIEHS), I was told, "The genomics revolution is washing over us. Either we incorporate it or we'll be left behind" (Field Notes July 2002).

Incorporating molecular genomic research into the environmental health sciences would be no small task. Physicians long had deployed a variety of ideas about heredity in their explanations of health and disease (Rosenberg 2007). However, within public health, both research and interventions focused on factors *external* to the human body as the most critical causes of disease. As we have seen, one way that public health practitioners defined their jurisdiction (vis-à-vis medicine) was by maintaining a focus on the relationships among environments, bodies, and the health of the population. Through this professional division of labor, preventing disease by intervening in the environment became the domain of public health practitioners, whereas medical doctors treated individual patients in the clinic (Nash 2006). The environmental health sciences, on the whole, have been oriented to a public health approach focused on the population, rather than on individuals.

How, then, did environmental health scientists develop research agendas that allowed them to incorporate genetics while maintaining their focus on how the environment affects human health? This chapter traces the development of one of the two primary strategies used by environmental health scientists to put molecular genetics and genomics at the center of their work: environmental health research focused on *inherited genetic susceptibilities*, that is, genetic variations that make some people more vulnerable than others to harm from environmental exposures. This research constitutes one meaning of gene-environment interaction and is typified in the following statement: "The study of interaction between the environment and genetics . . . has identified variations in human genes which, under certain environmental exposures, increase the risk of acquiring cancer" (Simmons & Portier 2002: 903). In this definition of gene-environment interaction, environmental health scientists maintain a focus on the harmful effects of environmental contaminants, but they define variations in individuals' responses to contaminants as a crucial problem to be explained.[2]

In establishing this line of research, environmental health scientists molecularized broad concepts of constitutional difference, vested them in specific classes of genes, and made claims about the relevance of these genes both within and beyond the clinic. This chapter begins by briefly considering the historical meanings of constitutional concepts developed by medical practitioners—such as hypersensitivity, idiosyncrasy, and disease diathesis—that have been reanimated in contemporary research on genetic susceptibility to environmental exposures. It then traces the development of the concept of *chemical individuality*, especially in the fields of pharmacogenetics and ecogenetics, which provided environmental health scientists with a specific, molecular focus arguably relevant to their jurisdiction. The second half of the chapter centers on the Environmental Genome Project (EGP), an effort to identify and characterize genes that contribute to inter-individual variation in response to environmental exposures. It examines particularly how the institutional mandate of the NIEHS and the jurisdictional concerns of its scientists have shaped their efforts to define the environmental genome. Finally, the chapter examines how environmental health scientists make the case for the applications of environmental genomics research in both regulatory and clinical contexts, attending especially to the consequences of these applications for environmental biopolitics.

CONSTITUTIONAL CONCEPTS

Environmental health scientists certainly were not the first to propose that humans differ in our susceptibility to disease and our responses to medical treatments. Historically, concern about susceptibility derived primarily from clinical practice and research, where physicians and scientists proposed a number of concepts to capture the dimensions of what they called the "differential reactivity" and "essential inequality" of human bodies (Mendelsohn 2001; Rosenberg 2007).[3] For example, *predisposition* functioned as an operational concept that allowed bacteriologists to explain the differential outcomes of experimental infections in bacteriological testing. Bacteriological research also identified variations in how people responded to treatments. In 1893, Behring, a German physiologist, coined the term *hypersensitivity* to describe the condition of those who had adverse reactions to serum injections that did not cause harm in others. Although pharmacological and toxicological study had long provided evidence of *idiosyncrasy*, whereby some individuals evinced unusually intensive reactions to doses of serum, Behring advanced the notion that hypersensitivities designated not just exaggerated reactions, but also modes of specific predisposition to disease. Many physiologists believed it to be a fundamental law that "it is the organism and not the microbe that makes the disease" (Mendelsohn 2001: 32). Thus, even when Koch's pathogen was identified as the cause of tuberculosis, physicians continued to refer to constitutional concepts to explain differential susceptibility to it (Rosenberg 2007).

At the same time, physicians and scientists used the concept of *hereditary predisposition* to account for why not all of the children of parents with purportedly heritable conditions (e.g. gout, scrofula, insanity) would inherit their parents' disease. According to this model, individuals inherited not the disease itself but the potential for it, a *disease diathesis*, which could be triggered by environmental stimuli. Further, physicians maintained that diatheses were lodged deeply within the organized structures of the body and difficult to remove. Thus, the notion of diathesis provided physicians with a rationale for why their recommended treatment regimens did not relieve diseases in all persons. In fact, doctors often used the terms *heritable* and *incurable* as synonyms. Again, these concepts functioned as an account for bodily variation, both in regard to susceptibility to illness and response to available treatment modalities (Rosenberg 2007; Waller 2002b).

Then, as now, physicians' configurations of bodily differences had implications for how they understood the effects of "unfavorable environments" on human health. Writing in 1938, British geneticist J.B.S. Haldane argued that individual "constitution" was an important "side" of understanding—and possibly preventing—respiratory diseases among potters:

> But while I am sure that our standards on industrial hygiene are shamefully low, it is important to realize that there is a side to this question that has been completely ignored. The majority of potters do not die of bronchitis. It is quite possible that if we really understood the causation of this disease, we should find that only a fraction of potters are of a constitution that rendered them liable to it. . . . There are two sides to most of these questions involving unfavorable environments. Not only could the environment be improved, but susceptible individuals could be excluded . . . (Haldane 1938: 102).

Even committed constitutionalists debated whether bodily inequalities were primarily inherited, acquired (via the environment), or a combination of inherited and acquired traits. Many physicians believed that constitution was a blend of the influence of heredity and the environment (Rosenberg 2007: 102). Although diathesis was lodged deep within the body, the manifestation of illness (or its absence) was contingent on the interactions between the body and its environments. Additionally, the concept of hereditary predisposition explicitly highlighted the role of environmental factors in disease causation. In fact, some physicians used it to develop an extreme environmentalist position, arguing that "if precipitating factors are deemed necessary for the activation of hereditary taints, is it not just as reasonable to assume that these environmental causes are a sufficient condition for developing the illness?" (Waller 2002a: 422).[4]

There are clear conceptual continuities in these concerns about the relationships between heredity, the environment, and human health and illness, as well as current articulations of gene-environment interaction. However, how scientists actually measure heredity and study the effects of the environment have changed dramatically. Early notions of predisposition had no ontology; physicians saw heredity as a process that unfolded over time, rather than as a discrete mechanism (Mendelsohn 2001: 30; Rosenberg 2007: 102). In contrast, contemporary research on susceptibility focuses on specific genes at the molecular level.

CHEMICAL INDIVIDUALITY: METABOLISM
IN THE CLINIC AND BEYOND

For environmental health scientists, mid- to late twentieth-century research on genetic variations in metabolism provided the material and conceptual bridge to contemporary, molecular understandings of genetic susceptibilities to environmental pollutants. The concept of *inborn errors of metabolism* was proposed first by British physician and scientist Sir Archibald Garrod (Childs 1970). Based on studies of familial conditions, such as alcaptonuria and albinism, Garrod demonstrated that certain hereditary[5] disorders were caused by "deficiencies" in enzymes involved in metabolism (1901; 1902; 1909). Garrod was especially interested in "the differences in type which are so important in . . . the idiosyncrasies with regard to drugs and food," which he believed to underlay "the proverbial saying that what is one man's meat is another man's poison" (1909: 3). Insofar as inborn errors of metabolism caused individuals to have different responses to ingested substances, Garrod argued, they provided evidence of human "chemical individuality" (1902).

In his later writings, Garrod explicitly connected the concept of chemical individuality with constitutional predisposition, commenting, for example, that "I, for one, believe that the liabilities of certain individuals to, or their immunity from, certain maladies—what may be called their diatheses—have chemical origins" (quoted in Childs 1970: 72). He also proposed connections between predispositions, chemical individuality, and molecules: "[T]he factors which confer upon us our predispositions to and immunities from the various mishaps that are spoken of as diseases, are inherent in our very chemical structure; and even in the molecular groupings which confer upon us our individualities and from which we sprang" (quoted in Childs 19070: 73). Garrod's focus on the chemical basis of constitutional differences provided a bridge from research, in which constitution (or diathesis) was seen as a general property of families or individuals, to research, in which disease susceptibility could be thought of "in terms of the molecule" (quoted in Childs 1970: 72).[6]

In the decades immediately following Garrod's research and writing, inborn errors of metabolism were studied primarily by scientists interested in exploring patterns of Mendelian inheritance. Many of the outcomes of the errors under study were of limited clinical relevance (e.g., variations in capacity to taste or smell particular substances); they were compelling to scientists primarily as a means of investigating genetics in human populations (Weber 2001). However, during the Second World War, inborn errors of metabolism, and associated susceptible phenotypes, emerged as a subject of systematic clinical and scientific concern (Jensen 1962).[7]

During World War II, as part of preparing soldiers for combat overseas, military doctors gave antimalarial drugs to thousands of men in the American and British armies. Administering drugs to such a large population made it possible for military doctors to observe that a proportion of those receiving antimalarial drugs experienced "serious untoward side effects," especially acute hemolytic anemia (Jensen 1962). Researchers were particularly intrigued by what they believed to be racial variation in these responses, noting that "pamaquine caused hemolysis in 5–10% of American Negroes [sic] but rarely in Caucasians," among the U.S. servicemen; likewise, it was more prevalent among the Indian, Israeli, and Greek men serving in the British army (Tarlov et al. 1962: 214). The U.S. Army and the Office of the Surgeon General provided funding to the University of Chicago Army Malaria Research Unit to identify the basis of this adverse response and to chart its clinical course (Dern et al. 1954; Beutler et al. 1954).

Research on hemolytic response to antimalarial compounds was undertaken using prisoners in the Illinois State Penitentiary, who were given the drugs and then closely observed by researchers.[8] In their notes, the researchers observed that hemolytic crisis "is a phenomena almost exclusively limited to a few susceptible members of heavily pigmented races"[9] and concluded that "the drug induced hemolytic reaction occurring in primaquine sensitive subjects is due to a unique susceptibility of the red blood cell . . . " (Dern et al. 1954). They also demonstrated that this injury to red blood cells (and subsequent hemolytic anemia) was the same as that suffered by sensitive individuals when they ate fava beans or were exposed to certain industrial chemicals and dyes (Jensen 1962: 212). In 1956, the scientists identified the "major known enzymatic defect in primaquine sensitive individuals" to be glucose-6-phosphate dehydrogenase (G6PD) deficiency (Carson et al. 1956). In subsequent research, scientists demonstrated showed that G6PD deficiency is "a genetically transmitted *inborn error of metabolism*" and described both the mode of inheritance and distribution of the trait (Tarlov et al. 1962, emphasis added).

Scientists used G6PD research to highlight the power of new scientific methods to molecularize constitutional concepts such as idiosyncrasy and hypersensitivity by identifying precise mechanisms of susceptibility. From their perspective, G6PD provided "an example of a disease which, in the past, was looked upon as a reaction of idiosyncratic nature or as a hypersensitivity phenomenon and which is now better defined in terms of genetic abnormality and biochemical mediation of disease" (Jensen 1962: 212). As a consequence of this work, idiosyncrasies and hypersensitivities were identified as *molecular* phenomena that scientists could study and explain using the tools of genetics and biochemistry.

At about the same time that American scientists characterized the G6PD deficiency, researchers in Canada demonstrated that genetic control of a drug-metabolizing enzyme, n-acetyltransferase, was responsible for clinical variations in response to procainamide, a local anesthetic that caused prolonged apnea and death in some patients (Kalow 1968). This research established that *differences* in metabolizing enzymes, as well as metabolic disorders (such as G6PD), could cause individuals to have unique and adverse responses in response to pharmaceuticals (Kalow, personal communication, 2001). Building on this insight, scientists proceeded to identify genetic control of drug metabolism as the source of serious adverse reactions to a variety of drugs (Calabrese 1984). They called this domain of inquiry *pharmacogenetics*.

Early research in pharmacogenetics focused on the resistance of microorganisms and insects to drugs and insecticides, human genetic conditions with consequences for drug toxicities, purportedly racial differences in drug metabolism and, most broadly, genetic control of drug metabolism (Evans 1963; Kalow 1962; Meier 1963). In much of this early research, scientists endeavored to use drug response as an opportunity to reveal patterns of human genetic variation. Reflecting this focus, in the first review article of the field, published in the *Journal of the American Medical Association* in 1963, Evans defined pharmacogenetics as "the study of genetically determined variations that are revealed solely by the effects of drugs" (1963: 639). [10]

FROM PHARMACOGENETICS TO ECOGENETICS

Although the focus of pharmacogenetics is on clinical interventions (and their consequences), the concepts and practices of pharmacogenetics provided the conceptual and material resources with which scientists began to conceptualize and investigate genetic susceptibilities to *environmental* exposures. In 1957, Arno Motulsky, an American geneticist, noted that the individual variations observed in response to drugs might be related to susceptibility or resistance to conditions other than "drug idiosyncrasies": ". . . genetically conditioned drug reactions not only are of practical significance, but may be considered pertinent models for demonstrating the interaction of heredity and environment in the pathogenesis of disease" (Motulsky 1957: 836). Early extensions of pharmacogenetics focused especially on the workplace, with occupational hygienists using the tools of pharmacogenetics to identify susceptibilities to industrial chemicals (Stokinger 1962; Zavon 1962; Jensen 1962). For example, industrial hygienists used a model developed in studies of the relationship between G6PD deficiency and hemolytic anemia to investigate genetic susceptibility to two air pollutants, ozone and nitrogen dioxide (Mountain 1963: 360). Similarly, researchers used sensitivity to isoniazid, an antibiotic used to treat tuberculosis, to demonstrate the relevance of a particular form of metabolism (n-acetylation) in the detoxification and excretion of environmental exposures (Schulte & Perera 1993: 282). The interest of industrial hygienists in genetic susceptibility was not limited to the advancement of scientific understanding. Rather, as noted in an early publication, "The industrial physician could employ to advantage such tests *to distinguish heredity based disease from job claimed disability*" (Stokinger, Mountain, & Scheel 1968: 973, emphasis added).[11]

Building on the research of industrial hygienists, scientists argued that pharmacogenetics revealed only "the first tip of the iceberg" of a much broader set of susceptibilities to environmental exposures: "[F]rom our knowledge of genetic variability and pharmacogenetics, we can be sure that other pollutants are even now finding genetically susceptible targets . . . " (Brewer 1971: 93). Indeed, although it is common practice to differentiate between chemicals we ingest intentionally (e.g., drugs) and those to which we are exposed involuntarily (e.g., environmental pollutants), scientists demonstrated that the basic physiological processes of metabolism and excretion of these chemicals are often shared. Based on these observations, scientists coined the term *ecogenetics* to refer more broadly to such susceptibilities: "we used and promoted the term *ecogenetics* and applied it to a whole array of things . . . for pharmaceuticals, for environmental chemicals, for diet and nutrition, for allergens and food additives, for risk of infectious agents . . . all of that comes together in what we call ecogenetics, and that was really mobilized in the early 70's" (Interview S09). Ecogenetic researchers thus expanded the focus of research on genetic control of the metabolism of chemicals beyond the clinic, to the factory and the community, domains under the jurisdiction of public health research, practice, and policy making.

Throughout the 1970s and early 1980s, environmental health scientists considered ecogenetics at conferences (Omenn & Gelboin 1983) and in their publications (Calabrese 1984). In 1975, a report by the National Academy of Sciences featured a separate section on the role of genetic metabolic errors as predisposing factors in the development of toxicity from occupational *and* environmental pollutants. An appendix to the report listed 92 "genetic disorders" that research suggested could predispose affected persons to the toxic effects of pollutants (NAS 1973/1975: 337–339). In the late 1980s and early 1990s, the Schools of Public Health at the University of Cincinnati and the University of Washington established Centers for Ecogenetics, formally institutionalizing ecogenetic concerns within the jurisdiction of public health.

The response of the regulatory agencies, however, was equivocal. In 1978, an EPA conference was held on high-risk groups and pollutants that included a major section on genetic factors. That year, the EPA began to require that contractors writing health effects documents include in their reports to the Agency consideration of the effects of the chemical agent in question on "persons at higher-than-normal risk" (Calabrese

1986: 1098). However, the EPA definition of high-risk groups focused on gender, age, and morbidities, such as respiratory illnesses; genetic variations in susceptibility to environmental exposures were not mandated as a focus of environmental risk assessment or regulation.

Consequently, in the mid-1990s, when the NIEHS decided to make susceptibility to environmental exposures a research priority for the environmental health sciences, researchers were well aware that individuals and subpopulations vary in their susceptibilities to environmental exposures. However, environmental health scientists tended to view these variations as an "annoyance" and used methods, in both human and animal studies, to minimize their effect (Hattis 1996). Likewise, genetic susceptibility to environmental exposures did not have a formal role in processes of environmental health risk assessment and regulation (Smith 1996). With the EGP, the NIEHS endeavored to move research on genetic susceptibilities from the margins to the center of environmental health science and to establish a role for environmental genomic knowledge in the governance of environmental health and illness.

DISCOVERING ENVIRONMENTAL RESPONSE GENES

In 1997, the NIEHS announced the launch of the EGP.[12] The rationale for the project was that "the key to understanding how [environmental] agents lead to disease in diverse populations, and to gauging susceptibility in communities at large, may lie in common genetic differences, or polymorphisms" (NIEHS 1997). The goals of the EGP included (1) to identify allelic variants (polymorphisms) in *environmental disease susceptibility genes,* (2) to develop a central database for these genes, and (3) to foster population-based studies of gene-environment interaction in disease etiology. [13] Towards these ends, the EGP was to undertake resequencing of 200 environmental disease susceptibility genes in samples from 1,000 individuals. The resequencing effort was also essential to the overarching mission of the Project, which proposed the identification of the *environmental genome,* a concept developed by the NIEHS leadership, and investigation of its effects in population-based studies (Olden, Guthrie, & Newton 2001: 1966).[14]

In defining the environmental disease susceptibility genes at the center of the EGP, NIEHS scientists drew on theories and methods from pharmacogenetics and ecogenetics.[15] For example, they asserted that "genetic variability in several super-families of xenobiotic metabolizing enzymes (e.g., cytochrome P450s, glutathione-S-transferases, and N-acetyltransferases) is the major determinant of host-specific chemical susceptibility" (Olden, Guthrie, & Newton 2001: 1966). As noted, as early as the 1960s, occupational hygienists had begun to apply pharmacogenetics in nonclinical contexts by looking at the function of drug-metabolizing enzymes in response to occupational and environmental exposures. In the early 1990s, environmental health scientists extended this work, reconceptualizing drug-metabolizing enzymes as "carcinogen-metabolizing enzymes" and investigating their role in shaping responses to environmental contaminants:

> We were interested in whether drug metabolizing enzymes—*or, as we renamed them, carcinogen metabolizing enzymes*—were important modifiers of response to environmental exposures. And we had some early successes. We were able to explain the idea of genetics modifying environmental responses (Field Notes, NIEHS 2002, emphasis added).

As one scientist put it, "We picked up that concept. Because if it were true for drugs, which are really just beneficial chemicals, than why wouldn't it be true for environmental chemicals?" (Interview S29).

Among these successes of this approach was research by NIEHS scientists Doug Bell and Jack Taylor, which demonstrated that specific genetic polymorphisms that control enzymes involved in the metabolism of carcinogens (*NAT1, NAT2* and *GSTM*) are associated with an increased risk of bladder cancer among smokers (Bell et al. 1993). This research was the first study to show that specific genetic polymorphisms controlling the metabolism of an environmental exposure (e.g., chemicals in cigarettes) can raise the risk of cancer in humans (Manuel 1996). Their work thereby provided the proof of principle for the EGP, establishing the feasibility and potential importance of research to identify polymorphisms that modify responses to environmental exposures.

Although such research made genes controlling xenobiotic metabolism the "easiest to deal with" in the context of the EGP (Guengerich 1998: 367), NIEHS scientists did not want the EGP to be limited to these genes. At the time that the EGP was launched, scientists were expecting to find that there were as many as 100,000 genes in the human genome,[16] which posed the question, "which of these are environmental disease susceptibility genes?" In an article announcing the launch of the EGP, the NIEHS noted that "with only 200 genes to be sequenced . . . deciding on the most appropriate methods for selecting the test genes may take some time" (EHP 1997). Indeed, the sample size for the project was immediately contested (Loffredo, Silbergeld, & Parascandola 1998).

The NIEHS leadership met these challenges with both conceptual and procedural strategies. First, they proposed broad categories of potential genetic foci, based on the schema of pathways shown in Figure 2 that lead from environmental exposure to human biological response and, potentially, to disease outcomes. Thus, scientists conceptualized environmental disease susceptibility genes as *all* those genes involved in molecular mechanisms of the human body's response to environmental exposures. This included not only genes involved in metabolism and detoxification (i.e., the foci of earlier pharmacogenetic and ecogenetics research), but also hormone metabolism genes, receptor genes, DNA repair genes, cell cycle genes, cell death control genes, genes mediating immune and inflammatory responses, genes mediating nutritional factors, genes involved in oxidative processes, and genes for signal transduction systems (Environmental Genome Project website, accessed September 1999). The concept of *environmental response machinery* provided a mechanistic logic to the notion of environmental disease susceptibility by pointing to genes along specific molecular pathways. Concomitantly, scientists began to use the phrase *environmental response genes* to describe the focus of the EGP.

Second, the NIEHS asked what it called "the general scientific community" for nominations for candidate genes to be resequenced as part of the EGP. A candidate gene submission form was available on the first iteration of the EGP website. Visitors to the website could also view the

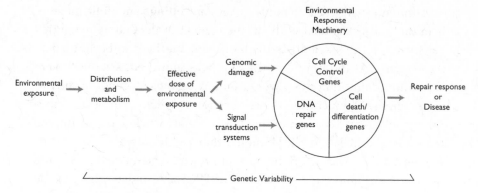

Figure 2. Genetic variability in response to environmental exposure.
Source: NIEHS (1997).

candidate gene list, which provided the names of genes that had been nominated by other scientists. This candidate gene list was then peer reviewed by a working committee of approximately 30 geneticists, epidemiologists, and policy makers, who were also charged with establishing a study group to provide peer review for all aspects of the project. The NIEHS's candidate gene approach balanced a relatively open and participatory selection process—one in which anyone could nominate a gene for resequencing—with scientific peer review, the gold standard for rigor and objectivity in science (Timmermans & Berg 1997). Based on these recommendations, NIEHS identified 554 environmentally responsive genes to be resequenced in the EGP (Wakefield 2002).

As I detail in the following pages, the NIEHS was committed to differentiating the EGP from the Human Genome Project and private sector efforts focused on gene discovery; the candidate gene approach served this purpose, as well. The summary of the 1997 Environmental Genome Project symposium stated specifically that "*this will not be a gene discovery project*" but rather "will exploit information provided by the U.S. Department of Energy and the Human Genome Institute's *gene-identification*" (NIEHS 1997, emphasis added). The goals of exploiting information from the Human Genome Project and making it relevant to the environmental health sciences were institutionalized as criteria that the peer review committee used to prioritize genes for resequencing. Preference was given to genes "not only whose sequence is known but, more importantly, to those implicated for their role in environmentally-associated diseases" and for which there was extant knowledge regarding gene structure, function, and interactions (NIEHS 1997). The scientific rationale for these selection criteria was that because "the candidate genes are fairly well characterized and in most cases have a significant probability of playing a role in disease susceptibility, the SNPs identified by the EGP have a good chance of being functionally important" (Wilson & Olden 2004: 150).[17] However, positioning the EGP as the "second generation of the Human Genome Project" (Olden & Guthrie 2001: 6) was also important to the efforts of the NIEHS to differentiate the EGP from the genomics initiatives of other Institutes.

INSTITUTIONALIZING ENVIRONMENTAL GENOMICS

Jurisdictional concerns and institutional relationships at the National Institutes of Health profoundly shaped the definition of environmental disease susceptibility genes, the environmental response machinery, and, consequently, the environmental genome. In their initial conceptualization of environmental disease susceptibility genes as "functionally important variations in DNA sequence, common polymorphisms, in known genes that are likely to be influenced by environmental exposures," NIEHS scientists deliberately drew a distinction between genes that "act predominantly on their own to cause disease," which were at the center of the Human Genome Project, and genes "that act in concert with environmental agents," which they positioned as uniquely the focus of the EGP (NIEHS 1997, emphasis added). In publications announcing the EGP, the NIEHS highlighted the difference between its focus on environmental disease susceptibility genes and the initiatives of the National Human Genome Research Institute (NHGRI) and National Cancer Institute (NCI), which focused on "disease genes" (EHP 1997: 1298). Likewise, the EGP website stated in bold font that the EGP is **not** a part of the NHGRI's Human Genome Project, positioning it rather as part of the mission of the NIEHS:

> The Environmental Genome Project was conceived by NIEHS scientists as a means to *further advance the mission of the NIEHS. This is very different from the Human Genome Project.* While relying heavily on the technology developed by the Human Genome Project, the Environmental Genome Project plans to determine sequence variation of environmental response genes; i.e. genes that determine susceptibility to environmentally induced diseases (Environmental Genome Project website, accessed September 1999).

In scientific publications as well, NIEHS scientists drew distinctions between genes that cause disease and the focus of the EGP on genes that modify risk following environmental exposures (Olden & Guthrie 2001: 5).

Such distinctions both reflected and reinforced the jurisdiction of the NIEHS within the institutional context of the National Institutes of Health. The Institute's leadership believed that a NIEHS genomics initiative that did not focus on environmental exposures would be seen by their colleagues as inappropriate to the NIEHS mission and an incursion on the "turf" of other Institutes:

> At the Institute, we *have to be concerned with potential overlap with other institutions. We have to separate our turf from that of the other Institutes.* The two words that do that are "environmental" and "toxicology." With this initiative [the Environmental Genome Project], we wanted to use the word "genome" but also separate our work from National Human Genome Research Institute. But then also, to build on the success of the Human Genome Project, to bring genomics into our field, to be nice and linear, within the context of the NIH and of such *institutional jurisdiction* (Interview S27, emphasis added).

The concept of environmental disease susceptibility genes provided both a focus and a rationale for a genomics initiative within the jurisdiction of the environmental health sciences. It allowed the EGP to incorporate genomics into environmental health research, without creating the perception that the NIEHS was attempting to encroach upon the domain of any other Institute. This was particularly important as several more well funded and powerful Institutes were starting genomics initiatives at the same time.

> Some institutes had parallel or related projects. At NHLBI [National Heart Lung and Blood Institute] they were studying genetic variation in relationship to blood pressure and stroke. And at NCI they were about to get a SNP project up and running (Interview S26).

At the same time, the environmental genome gave environmental health scientists their own "turf" in genomics research. Even scientists who questioned specifics of the EGP perceived it to be of strategic importance to the NIEHS vis-à-vis its stature at the NIH:

> In the mid 80's . . . they [NIEHS] were just falling behind completely, compared to the rest of NIH. . . . The institute was not getting as much money as it deserved . . . *there was a need to compete* with Francis Collins and the Human Genome Project . . . to do something relevant to environmental health that sounded like the Human Genome Project. So the Environmental Genome [Project] was a great idea from that point of view (Interview S20, emphasis added).

Indeed, the NIEHS leadership was eager to "get out in front" of efforts that might encroach on its focus on the environment and human health:

> And so we then rolled out a major national effort to identify all the genes in the human genome that make us more or less susceptible to environmental exposure . . . *we didn't want to trample on anybody else's territory, and so we said, those genes that make you more or less susceptible to environmental exposure.* Well there are predisposition genes that have nothing to do with the environment. And so, you know, NHGRI and all the other institutes can look at those. Of course, they can look at *ours* too. But the point is, we got out in front of that (Interview S37, emphasis added).

In fact, the NIEHS leadership hoped that the EGP would foster positive relationships—and new collaborations—between the NIEHS and other Institutes. In developing the EGP, NIEHS scientists made an effort to consult with the NIH leadership and with the directors of prestigious institutes, such as the NHGRI and the NCI:

> [We] did a big presentation at the NIH to Varmus, then the director of the NIH, Collins, the director of NHGRI, Klausner, the director of NCI, and Trent, the science director at NHGRI. They all were enthusiastic— thought that it was a great idea. So, in Fall of 1997, we had a symposium for the NIEHS community (Interview S26).

Reflecting on the symposium that launched the EGP, then NIEHS Deputy Director Samuel Wilson commented that "the symposium served to reinforce the NIEHS's working interactions with two of its sister institutions, the National Human Genome Research Institute and the National Institute of Cancer" (EHP 1997).

Related, NIEHS administrators contend that, with the launch of the EGP, the leadership of these Institutes "see how important our [NIEHS] work is for public health" (Field Notes, NIH December 2001). However, articulating the relevance of the EGP for environmental governance has raised thorny questions about the appropriate relationship between the biomedical orientation of research on genetic susceptibility and the population-level public health approaches that have long been at the center of environmental health governance.

RESPONDING TO ENVIRONMENTAL RESPONSE GENES

From the beginning of the EGP, NIEHS scientists have claimed that research on environmental response genes would have important public health applications. In a report on the symposium at which the EGP was announced, the deputy director of the NIEHS described the meeting as "an interesting and exciting scientific discussion on *the use of genomics to impact public health in the future*" (EHP 1997, emphasis added). NIEHS authors contended that the EGP would "revolutionize the practice of public health as it relates to environmental health protection" (Olden, Guthrie, & Newton 2001: 1966). Even skeptics of the Project noted that "genetics has increasingly become, like epidemiology, as much a tool for public health as

a scientific discipline . . . improving public health is the primary goal . . . "
(Loffredo, Silbergeld, & Parascandola 1998: 368). However, scientists promulgated varied roles for environmental genomic knowledge. On the one
hand, environmental health scientists argued that environmental genomics
research had the potential to improve risk assessment and thereby refine
environmental regulation and policy making. At the same time, scientists
articulated a role for environmental susceptibility genes in the clinic.

Governing Susceptibilities

As detailed in Chapter 2, in promoting a role for molecular genetic and
genomic techniques in their research, environmental health scientists
point to variation in susceptibility as one of the intractable problems in
the risk assessment process (Olden, 2002: 275). Related, in their advocacy
for environmental genomics, NIEHS scientists claimed, "To have intel-
ligent environmental regulatory policy, one has to begin to unravel the
role of genetics in determining the differences in susceptibility" (Kaiser
1997). More dramatically, in a 1997 article in *Environmental Health Perspectives*, NIEHS Director Olden warned, "There may be an average exposure, but not an average individual . . . *whether we're actually protecting
the health of the American people is uncertain*. We may be under-regulating
or over-regulating" (Albers 1997, emphasis added). The possibility that
the EGP would refine regulatory processes, observed one science writer,
was "music to the ears of members of Congress who have been clamor-
ing for better science behind regulations" (Kaiser 1997). Indeed, speaking
before Congress in support of his proposed budget for fiscal year 2002,
Olden argued for the importance of environmental genomic research to
policy making:

> Presently, environmental health regulatory agencies craft rules as if
> "one-size-fits-all." However, we know that individuals can vary by more
> than two-thousand fold in their capacity to repair or prevent damage
> following exposure to toxic agents in the environment. *Knowledge of
> the prevalence of susceptibility genes would take much of the guesswork out
> of environmental health decision-making* (Olden, Fiscal Year 2002 Budget
> Statement, emphasis added).

At the same time, scientists were somewhat circumspect in their critiques of risk assessment, claiming that environmental regulations did "a pretty good job given the data that are available" but would be improved by environmental genomic research (Albers 1997).

Environmental health scientists identify three broad ways that data about susceptibilities to environmental exposures could be incorporated into analyses of the risks posed by specific chemicals. First, information about polymorphisms could be integrated into models that describe the absorption, distribution, metabolism, and elimination (ADME) of specific chemicals:

> If I know a particular enzyme that is polymorphic that alters the metabolism, I ought to be able to enter that directly into my model. If I know the percentage of the population that has that polymorphism and I'm trying to estimate population risks, I can adjust and do two models; one for this percent of the population, one for that percent, and then the actual population risk is the weighted average between the two. Really straightforward and simple. If it is two genes, so be it. My model has to include the two genes and the interactions between the two genes. If it's fifty genes I don't care, as long as I include them in the model . . . (Interview S41).

However, as he continued, "The way most people want to use environmental genomics is the other way around," that is, in epidemiological studies.

Multiple researchers at NIEHS and beyond told me that the "real goal" (Field Notes, NIEHS 2002) and "next challenge" (Interview S93) for the EGP was integrating data about polymorphisms into epidemiology. For example, data about environmental response genes could be used to "split" the population under study, so that the effects of a chemical exposure could be assessed separately in people with and without a specific genetic susceptibility (Interview S43). This could increase the sensitivity of environmental epidemiological studies, thereby enabling the identification of associations between exposure and illness that otherwise would not be identified in studies of the general population:

> So . . . you can argue that if there are genes that modify the health effects, we don't really understand the health effects well without trying to measure genetic polymorphisms. So for example, you know, we know that

asbestos causes lung cancer, but if we don't deal with cigarette smoking, our estimates of the risk are confounded by cigarette smoking. Similarly, if there is a subgroup who are working with lead who are at much greater risk for the health effects of lead, then we can underestimate the risk in that group if we don't account for their genetic variability (Interview S11).

To the extent that this approach enables environmental epidemiologists to identify the effects of exposures—even if only in specific subpopulations—scientists believe that it could contribute greatly to efforts to characterize the health risks of chemicals in the environment.

Lastly, data about environmental response genes could be used "to create a transgenic or knockout animal" as a model system for studying specific gene-environment interactions (Interview S80).[18] Genetically modified animal models, in turn, could provide a means of investigating the effects of human genes in gene-environment interactions (e.g., Medina et al. 2002):

> If I suspect the gene is part of this problem in a human population, I can turn it on, turn it off, or modify its regulation in a genetically altered animal, and then do my cancer study. . . . The genetic modifications [shows] whether or not this gene/chemical interaction is important in a rodent population and potentially important in a human population . . . (Interview S41).

Modifications to animal models might also increase the sensitivity and specificity of cancer bioassays (Pritchard et al. 2003; Tennant, French, & Spalding 1995). All of these approaches are receiving funding as part of the next phases of the EGP (Wilson & Olden 2004: 150).

These applications of data about genetic susceptibilities to environmental health governance are revolutionary insofar as they introduce a new set of molecular techniques and foci into the risk assessment process. Further, these approaches work together to shift risk assessment techniques from animal models to human bodies. These are consequential changes. Indeed, in claiming that there is no average individual, environmental health scientists advocating for the inclusion of genetic susceptibilities in risk assessment have undermined the heuristic "standard human" that has been the subject of environmental risk assessment and policy making (Smith 1996; see also Epstein 2007).

However, these proposed applications maintain the longstanding relationships between the NIEHS and the EPA; the environmental health sciences would continue to serve as a source of empirical research that can serve as an evidence base for environmental policy making. Likewise, although these techniques make use of molecular genetic and genomic data, they do not require the identification of specific individuals at risk, as this molecular epidemiologist emphasized:

> Just because it involves genetics and environmental research doesn't mean you're doing genetic screening. If the research . . . shows that a very substantial percentage of the population is particularly vulnerable to, say, benzene or something, then the regulation would be to lower the permissible exposure limit to benzene for everyone, and would not require any sort of assessment of genotype . . . Presumably the research would have been done on risk populations representative of the U.S . . . they would then get translated into this legislation, and it would mean altering the standards, probably downward. I wouldn't see legislation requiring any type of genotyping or screening (Interview S06).

What is governed, according to this approach, is *the environment*. In contrast, environmental health scientists have suggested also that research on genetic susceptibility to environmental exposures would improve public health by making possible new forms of prevention and treatment (Guengerich 1998), in the form of a variety of clinical and lifestyle interventions targeted to genetically susceptible individuals.

Environmental Response Genes in the Clinic

As environmental health scientists advocated for increased attention to genetic susceptibilities in the risk assessment process, they realized that, even if their efforts were successful, "we still would have a problem: how do you use that information on the individual level?" (Interview S13). Put differently, as environmental genomic research began to identify genes that make individuals and subpopulations particularly susceptible to the harmful effects of environmental exposures, scientists began to confront issues regarding whether identifying people at risk should have a role beyond environmental health research and risk assessment. Simply put, "the Environmental Genome Project does . . .

tell us . . . you can look at genetically sensitive individuals" (Interview S41). That is, it identifies a new category of human subjects—persons genetically susceptible to environmental exposures. Proposals regarding the use of environmental genomic knowledge to identify persons genetically at risk of being harmed by environmental exposures raise questions about the appropriate role of biomedicine in environmental governance.

In their articulations of the possibility of biomedical interventions based on environmental genomic research, NIEHS scientists often invoke the clinical encounter:

> . . . the answer to the most common question asked of physicians, i.e. "Why me, Doc? Why do I have lung cancer (berylliosis, asbestosis, asthma), whereas most of my associates who have had similar exposures have not developed these diseases?" will not be answered by looking only at the environment. One answer to these questions is that genetically-determined differences in susceptibility may be at least partly responsible (Olden & Guthrie 2001: 5).

This theme emerged also in interviews and observation at the NIEHS, with scientists asserting that their inspiration for undertaking environmental genomic research was to answer "the 'why me?' question" (Field Notes, NIEHS, 2002). Importantly, this framing shifts the focus of environmental research from the population level to the individual level and from the exposure to the gene. The question here is about the differential susceptibility of individuals, given similar exposures.

There are varied proposals, however, about what "doc" might do with knowledge about genetically determined differences in susceptibility to environmental exposures. These have included pharmacological treatment, gene therapy, and "lifestyle prescriptions" for those who are most susceptible. In articulating these possibilities, NIEHS scientists used the metaphor of a loaded gun to explain the relationship between genes and the environment: "A loaded gun by itself causes no harm; it is only when the trigger is pulled that the potential for harm is released or initiated. Likewise, one can inherit a predisposition for a devastating disease, yet never develop the disease unless exposed to the environmental trigger(s)" (Olden & Guthrie 2001: 3–4). From this perspective, "knowing whether or not one's genetic 'gun' is loaded can help one to avoid pulling the trigger" (Wilson & Olden 2000: 149). One proposal is that pharmacology might be used as prophylaxis to block the effects of a trigger:

> For example, what if we identified that someone is missing a certain enzyme. And exposure to a certain chemical in the water would cause them a problem. And that is something we can't get out of the water. Well, what about if that person were given a certain drug or certain dietary nutrients, which would now enable them to deal with that? In other words, I see a tremendous *therapeutic potential* (Interview P14, emphasis added).

Alternatively, NIEHS authors have proposed that individuals who are particularly susceptible to the harmful effects of chemicals might follow lifestyle prescriptions from their physicians:

> Knowledge of susceptibility will potentially change the "contract" between patient and physician from the current emphasis on curative treatment to prevention. The health care industry will have the information to sort the population into "bins" and prescribe a particular lifestyle for each group (Olden & Guthrie 2001: 8).

In these approaches, responsibility for preventing environmentally associated disease rests with individuals who are identified as members of "at-risk subpopulations" (EHP 1997), rather than with public policies to control environmental exposures. Consequently, though the EGP is framed as population-based research, it nonetheless is strongly oriented to interventions at the individual level.

Whether and when it is appropriate to deploy individual-level strategies, rather than public policy approaches, to prevent environmentally associated illnesses is a topic of controversy among environmental health scientists.[19] Some scientists contend that individual-level intervention will be necessary because public policy is not adequate to protecting the most susceptible members of the population. As this regulator stated, "It is difficult to regulate for the most susceptible person, the one in a million person" (Field Notes, WEACT 2002). Similarly, a former National

Toxicology Program (NTP) scientist emphasized the difficulty of "drawing the line" that determines for whom regulation will be sufficiently protective:

> The real difficult question comes in, how many people need to be sensitive before the government will step in to protect them? If there's one person in the world, then probably not . . . . Maybe 5% of the population? Yes, you protect them. But you also have to make it explicit that that's what your regulatory decision is based on. If it gets down to very low numbers, at some point you have to say, "No, we're not going to protect you" (Interview S81).

In contrast, some environmental health scientists have argued that because "genetic variants that confer risk to environmental toxins are innocuous in the absence of exposure to those toxins," removing toxins from the environment should remain the primary strategy of environmental governance (Field Notes, NIH 2001). Similarly, scientists contend that, given the relatively small effect of environmental response genes, "fundamentally" the issue is the exposure:

> So, even for an exposure like smoking, may be there are 5–10 things that put you at higher risk. But, fundamentally, smoking is the issue. And for exposures other than smoking, there's very little good data that points to any smoking guns (Interview S26).

Still other scientists propose that individual-level interventions might be important in situations when the environmental trigger cannot readily be removed from the environment. For example, former NIEHS Director Olden commented that:

> Our community thinks . . . you identify the risk factor and just remove it from the environment. But, there are a lot of environmental agents that we aren't going to be able to get out of the environment for a while (Olden, Oral History Interview July 2004).

As noted by Olden, this approach represents a move "beyond the status quo . . . [that is] we tell the EPA and FDA and OSHA and they regulate" (Olden, Oral History Interview July 2004).

At the same time, many scientists recognize the difficulty of translating environmental genomic information into public health interventions. Alongside standard ethical considerations, such as how to maintain the privacy of genetic information, environmental health scientists have raised concerns about the degree to which individuals can realistically be expected to act on information about genetic susceptibility to environmental toxicants. First, environmental health scientists note that individual-level, behavioral strategies represent a notoriously difficult way to improve population health. For example, though science has established that diet and nutrition powerfully shape health outcomes, "I talk to people on the diet side of all this, and they tell me it's nearly impossible to get people to change what they are eating" (Interview S26). Further, given that individuals are exposed to environmental chemicals in the places where they live, work, and play, effective interventions for susceptible individuals might require major life changes. As this toxicologist asked "So, what do we do when we know that people near a [contaminated] site are carrying this gene? Do we displace people from their work? From their land?" (Interview S29). A molecular epidemiologist argued that "there's no way you can screen people and have them move out of their communities. I think that's just over the top, ethically, and probably legally challengeable too" (Interview S06). A molecular epidemiologist who primarily studies exposure in the workplace concurred: "Well, if you can't exclude workers from the workplace on the basis of genetic information, then the only way we are going to be able to protect susceptible subgroups is by setting our permissible exposure limits lower. And so that is. . . . one of the potential benefits" (Interview S11).

Consequently, some observers of the EGP have argued against individual-level applications of environmental genomic data. Echoing analyses of the application of molecular genetic and genomic data in public health more broadly (Ottman 1995; cf. Khoury et al. 2000), they contend that the most effective disease prevention will result from intervention strategies aimed at *all* exposed individuals, rather than interventions only for genetically susceptible persons. Likewise, some environmental health scientists argue that disease prevention could be effectively accomplished by regulating the chemicals in the environment, independent of environmental genomic knowledge (Interview S96).

Reflecting on these two very different potential responses to environmental genomic knowledge, environmental health scientists have raised the question of whether environmental response genes are important to public health primarily as *confounding factors* in research that assesses environmental exposures and explicates the underlying mechanisms of toxicity (contributing to a more traditional public policy approach to environmental governance) or *as independent factors* that raise individual risk for adverse outcomes following environmental exposure (contributing to a clinical approach) (Field Notes, NIEHS 2002). Later genomics initiatives launched by the NIEHS, such as the collaborative Genes, Environment, and Health study announced in 2006, simultaneously pursue both strategies (Schwartz & Collins 2007).[20]

FROM THE ENVIRONMENT TO THE GENOME. . . AND BACK AGAIN?

The contemporary focus of environmental health scientists on individual and subpopulation susceptibility to environmental exposures gives new, molecular form to decades-old debates about whether individual bodily susceptibilities are relevant to public health policy and practice. The notion that "Genetics loads the gun, but it's the environment that pulls the trigger," often invoked by the NIEHS leadership in their advocacy of the EGP (Olden & Guthrie 2001; Olden & Wilson 2000), would not be a cause of controversy among nineteenth- and twentieth-century physicians. Albeit couched in the language of molecular genetics (and firearms), this notion is resonant with nineteenth- and early twentieth-century conceptualizations of unequal constitutions and disease diatheses. Assessing variations in individual disease risks and responses to treatment continues to be a defining focus of the contemporary biomedical sciences (Clarke et al. 2003). For example, understanding individual genetic susceptibility to disease, as well as individual response to pharmaceuticals, is at the center of human genome research (Guttmacher & Collins 2005). However, notions of constitution and predisposition have been marginal to, and often excluded entirely, from environmental health research and regulation (Hamlin 1992; Sellers 1997). As then NIEHS Director Olden noted in his testimony before Congress in 2001, environmental genomics' focus on individual (host) susceptibilities runs counter to the long-standing assumption in the environmental health sciences that "the dose makes the poison."

In making genetic susceptibilities to environmental exposures a focus of environmental health research, the NIEHS drew on conceptual and material resources from research on drug metabolism, pharmacogenetics, and ecogenetics. However, it also developed novel scientific work objects, such as the environmental genome, environmental response machinery, and environmental response genes, establishing them as new, molecular foci for environmental health research. With these new research foci, the NIEHS defined its institutional "turf" in the context of an array of NIH genomics research initiatives. At the same time, the NIEHS' focus on gene-environment interaction served as a means of building networks with other Institutes, including the NHGRI (Schwartz & Collins 2007). Thus, contemporary research on genetic susceptibility to environmental exposures, especially as manifest in the NIEHS's Environmental Genome Project, may be understood as an effort to both maintain and expand the jurisdiction of the environmental health sciences in the age of the genome. The expansionist aspirations of the NIEHS are perhaps most visible in efforts to develop uses for EGP research in individual-level, clinical settings, rather than solely as a basis for environmental health risk assessment and regulation. The potential of environmental genomics to inform *both* clinical and regulatory interventions means that it offers simultaneously a means of defending the traditional jurisdiction of the environmental health sciences and of opening the possibility of expansion.

How might we assess the outcomes of the EGP? One measure, featured prominently on the NIEHS website,[21] is to focus on the number of environmental response genes that have been resequenced. Specifically, the lead lab for the project, at the University of Washington, "has sequenced over 607 environmentally responsive genes in a panel of 95 human DNA samples. . . .They have sequenced in excess of 14 MB of baseline genome sequence, resulting in 85,547 SNPs."[22] Alternatively, one might evaluate the EGP's contribution to the data repository dbSNPs[23]: "NIEHS, through the efforts at the University of Washington, has been the fifth major producer of genotypes found in dbSNPs" (NIEHS EGP website; see also Livingston et al. 2004). Review articles have highlighted specific environmental response genes that scientists have characterized in research funded by the EGP (Wilson & Olden 2004). However, as with genomic research more broadly, the public health applications of environmental genomics remain "promissory" (Hedgecoe 2004). As noted in an article celebrating the fifth anniversary of the EGP, although the project is "advancing in step with it original goals of understanding the complex interrelationship between environmental exposure, genetic susceptibility, and human disease," EGP research "has been slow to trickle into the policy making arena" (Wakefield 2002: 758).

Members of the NIEHS leadership express great pride in the diffusion of the concept of gene-environment interaction across the NIH. In 2004, in an interview reflecting on his tenure as Director of the NIEHS, Olden commented "Francis Collins,[24] . . . he's very into [the] environment now . . . [he] uses the word "gene-environment interaction" as much as I do." Olden noted also that he had been invited to the five-year strategic planning meeting for the NHGRI, an invitation he attributed to the central role of gene-environment interaction to the emerging NHGRI agenda, which "can't go forward unless [they] understand the interactions" (Olden, Oral History Interview July 2004). The NIEHS and NHGRI now collaborate on two major NIH initiatives to understand gene-environment interactions in human development and common diseases, the National Children's Study and the Genes, Environment, and Health Initiative.

The role of the NIEHS in these collaborative research projects is to lead the "development of innovative technologies to measure environmental exposures (broadly defined) that contribute to the development of disease."[25] NIEHS administrators contend that the Institute's mandate to lead "Exposure Biology Programs" in each initiative is evidence that "the environment" is being recognized as "a major player" in human health and illness (Field Notes, NIEHS 2004). Moreover, they position these developments as concordant with the original goal of the EGP, " . . . to facilitate molecular epidemiology research in humans, *molecular in the sense of using exposure measurements, as well as genetic or DNA measure-ments"* (Interview S27, emphasis added). Thus, perhaps paradoxically, one consequence of research on genetic susceptibility to environmental exposures seems to be increased interest in *molecular measures of the environment*. An article describing the GEI (authored by former directors of the NIEHS and NHGRI) explicitly contrasted expenditures on genomics research with those for measuring environmental exposures:

> Progress in identifying genetic variations that contribute to common disease has been rapid in the last few years. The same rapid rate of progress has not been achieved for precise, quantitative assays to measure environmental factors that contribute to adverse health outcomes. Certainly, assessment of environmental contributions is much more difficult than for genetic ones. . . . *However, another explanation is apparent by contrasting the extensive investments in new genetic and genomic technologies over the past two decades with the much more modest expenditures in exposure sciences* (Schwartz & Collins 2007: 695, emphasis added).

In the following chapter, I consider how environmental exposures and their effects on human health are studied at the molecular level.

FOUR "Opening the Black Box of the Human Body"

> These are things we could never measure until now . . .
> Before, the body was like a big black box. We're finally
> getting inside the box.
>
> Dr. Frederica Perera[1]

The movement of knowledge production from cities, fields, and factories to the laboratory is a defining characteristic of the contemporary environmental health sciences.[2] Establishing the laboratory—rather than the actual locations where people live, work, and play—as a site of knowledge production about the relationships among bodies, the environment, and

Earlier versions of this analysis appeared in S. Shostak, "Marking Populations and Persons At Risk." In *Biomedicalization: Technoscience, Health, and Medicine in the U.S.* Edited by Adele E. Clarke, Laura Mamo, Jennifer Fosket, Jennifer Fishman, and Janet Shim. Durham, NC: Duke University Press. Copyright © 2010 Duke University Press; also in S. Shostak and E. Rehel. "Changing the Subject: Science, Subjectivity, and the Structure of 'Ethical Problems.'" In *Advances in Medical Sociology: Sociological Perspectives on Bioethical Issues.* Edited by Barbara Katz Rothman, Elizabeth Armstrong, and Rebecca Tiger. Oxford: Elsevier/JAI Press. Copyright © 2007 JAI/Emerald Press.

human health and illness poses enormous practical challenges. Specifically, it has required that scientists identify credible ways of representing the environment and modeling its effects on human bodies inside the space of the laboratory. Contemporary toxicologists meet such challenges primarily by measuring the effects of specific chemicals inside the bodies of highly standardized animal models. However, environmental epidemiologists, who seek to measure and characterize the effects of the environment within diverse human populations in complex and ever changing natural settings, face a different set of challenges. This chapter examines the efforts of environmental epidemiologists to use the tools of molecular biology to overcome the challenges facing their field. It describes particularly the development of molecular biomarkers as a means of measuring the environment at the molecular level and inside the human body.

The chapter begins by tracing the development of varied ways of conceptualizing the environment in two precursors of the contemporary environmental health sciences: sanitary engineering and industrial hygiene. I attend especially to the differences in scale at which each conceptualized the environment, the techniques of measurement deployed, and the aspects of the relationships between bodies and environments that were thereby rendered more or less visible.[3] These histories are used to contextualize the emergence of molecular epidemiology and its signal technology, molecular biomarkers. I position molecular biomarker techniques especially as a response to the unique challenges facing environmental epidemiology, which has been caught betwixt and between epidemiological, field-based approaches (developed within sanitary engineering), and toxicological, laboratory-based approaches (deriving from industrial hygiene) to studying the relationships between environmental exposures and human health. This "betweeness" has been especially problematic for environmental epidemiologists who, as a consequence, confront a unique set of vulnerabilities in establishing the credibility of their research. The chapter concludes with an extended case study of the use of molecular measures of the environment in an environmental health dispute in Midway Village, a public housing project in the San Francisco Bay Area. This case highlights the challenges of measuring the environment at the molecular level, assessing its relationships to human health, and developing effective interventions.

MEASURING ENVIRONMENTAL EXPOSURES

Lived Environments: Sanitation and Public Health

In the nineteenth century, public health reformers argued that miasma— principally filth and foul air—was responsible for outbreaks of infectious diseases that ravaged the population.[4] In Britain, the Sanitation Movement, led by Edwin Chadwick and his allies, focused research and policy efforts on eliminating "specific events that set a disease off, be they contagia, miasms, or something else" (Hamlin 1992: 44). Even as doctors argued that variation in individuals' responses to "the same noxious influence" made it impossible to attribute disease to environmental exposures alone, in both Britain and the United States, the Sanitarians endeavored to focus public health efforts on cleaning up the physical environment (Duffy 1992; Rosen 1993).

The Sanitarians' definition of the environment included what they called remote factors — for example, proper air, temperature, food, and exercise —that could strengthen or weaken individual constitutions, However, given the perceived difficulty of controlling remote factors, they focused their efforts primarily on the control of physical environments, emphasizing the importance of the "avoidance of poison" by reducing exposure to "filth" (Hamlin 1992: 66).[5] Their contemporary, Friedrich Engels, argued that the class structure of capitalism was at the root of the filthy conditions of the factories and neighborhoods where the poor worked and lived and that it must be redressed in order to improve the public's health (1844). However, even as they advocated for large-scale interventions, such as the construction of new public housing, sewer systems, paved streets, and sources of clean water for drinking and bathing, the Sanitarians refrained from blaming specific social or economic structures for the inequities and illnesses they sought to remedy (Corburn 2009: 29–30). In contrast with Engels, their interventions focused largely on what is now called "the built environment" rather than the social structures and processes that led to its particular forms.

In the 1900s, the Sanitarians' emphasis on keeping bodies and environments clean was carried forward in the work of sanitary engineering and public health. Despite the rise of the germ theory of disease—with its focus on individual pathogens and their pathways into the human body—public health efforts continued to seek to address the environment's role in disease. Indeed, as medicine focused increasingly on the clinical treatment of the individual, public health practitioners defined their jurisdiction, in part, by maintaining a focus on relationships among environments, bodies, and health. Sanitary engineers, in particular, focused on improvements to the physical design of both the urban neighborhoods and rural landscapes where people lived and worked. Their signal practice was the sanitary survey or inspection. In cities, the survey was an effort to describe every street, building, and lot within a given area in order to determine both the location of diseases and the environmental conditions that might give rise to them. City planners used data from sanitary surveys to guide interventions such as constructing new water supply and sewer systems, paving streets and wharves, destroying substandard housing, and developing parks. In rural and farming communities, field inspections conducted by sanitary engineers endeavored to identify and then eradicate environments that were likely to produce and sustain disease (Corburn 2009; Nash 2006).

Both the ethos of sanitary engineers and the public health interventions based on their work were progressive in that they assumed that urban and rural environments could be managed and reorganized to support human health. In cities like New York and Chicago, prominent social reformers, including Alice Hamilton and Florence Kelly, played key roles; their work included extended surveys of neighborhoods and factories (Sellers 1997). Sanitary engineering preserved a space of practice in which broad social and political conceptualizations of the environment could coexist with germ theory. Consequently, as new ways of knowing the environment—powerfully linked to the techniques of bacteriology—began to emerge, researchers concerned with the associations between the environment and human health were forced to consider their relationship not only to new laboratory techniques, but also to progressive politics.[6]

The Environment Inside: Industrial Hygiene, Occupational Health, and the Rise of Modern Toxicology

Although many contemporary environmental health scientists are proud to claim the Sanitary Movement as part of their professional lineage (e.g., Parodi, Neasham, & Vineis 2006) the laboratory-based practices of contemporary environmental health science, and especially toxicology, derive most directly from the field of industrial hygiene (Sellers 1997). In the first half of the twentieth century, industrial hygienists established laboratory and experimental techniques as a means of assessing and quantifying the relationship between bodies, environments, and human health and illness. Laboratory techniques were central to industrial hygienists' efforts to consolidate their professional power and establish their political independence, both from both the progressive movement and from the industries whose factories and workers they studied. Their successes in establishing laboratory models for studying exposures in the factory have profoundly shaped the practices—and the challenges—of contemporary environmental health science (Sellers 1997).

Industrial hygienists strategically distanced themselves from the reformist agenda of earlier modes of investigation, offering their professional scientific services to companies "as an objective, apolitical, and nonlegislative way to arbitrate occupational disease disputes" (Murphy 2006: 86). Central to their claim to expertise was the move from the factory to the laboratory and from human bodies to animal models. In addition to purportedly depoliticizing their science, shifting the location of the investigation out of the factory and into the lab provided researchers with a way of avoiding many practical challenges involved in studying the workplace itself. Whereas industrial hygienists associated with the Progressive Movement focused on public and industrial hygienic conditions, laboratory-based industrial hygienists focused their research on what the French physiologist Claude Bernard called the *milieu interieur*, or internal environment. That is, they focused *inside the body* and most often inside the bodies of the animals that increasingly "stood in" for humans in the lab (Sellers 1997: 161).

In addition to allowing them to sidestep many of the social, political, and practical challenges of studying the workplace, the shift to laboratory techniques focused on the *milieu interieur* gave industrial hygienists privileged access to a realm that was both inaccessible to parties to industrial disputes (e.g., workers, managers, and factory doctors) and firmly within the jurisdictions of medicine and science (Sellers 1997: 161). Indeed, industrial hygienists highlighted the "dependability" of laboratory techniques for identifying "what was invisible to the clinician or worker: the specific chain of effects that a chemical consistently caused in human physiology . . . " (Murphy 2006: 86–87). With the help of collaborators in physiology and chemistry, industrial hygienists conceptualized the body in terms of chemistry and chemical regulation and focused "inward, toward constituents and processes more thoroughly sealed within the *milieu interieur*" (Sellers 1997: 221).

In seeking to make good on its promise to provide objective descriptions of the causes and physiological characteristics of industrial disease by focusing inside the human body, industrial hygienists also instantiated specific conceptualizations and measurements of the environment. The laboratory and experimental techniques used by academic industrial hygienists borrowed heavily from bacteriological models of human bodies, health, and illness. The possibility of defining discrete and specific occupational diseases with singular chemical causes was particularly compelling to physicians and public health officials who had embraced germ theory. Consequently, in industrial hygiene labs—and, later, in toxicological research—the external environment was reinterpreted in "chemicophysical terms" and "reduced to a set of discrete chemicals" (Sellers 1997: 165; Nash 2006: 159). As with germ theory, the assumption was that disease was caused by a discrete entity that entered the body from the environment through specific, traceable pathways.

The move to the laboratory and researchers' increasing reliance on animal models provided also a means of minimizing the variability and complexity of environments and bodies that, outside the laboratory, were relatively less easily controlled or neatly quantified. Thus, the new science of industrial hygiene excluded not only the social, political, and economic contexts of environmental exposures, but also more complex environmental influences on human health and illness, such as chemical mixtures, chronic low-dose exposures, and the idiosyncrasies of individual exposure histories and bodily variations.[7]

In their attempts to understand the effects of the broader environment (i.e., beyond the workplace) on human health, modern toxicologists are the epistemic inheritors of early twentieth-century industrial hygiene. Toxicological research, in general, conceptualizes the environment in terms of single chemical agents, relies heavily on the use of animal models, seeks to define specific pathways of exposure, and focuses on contaminants that can be measured and identified in the laboratory. For example, the current gold standard of toxicology testing is the two-year rodent cancer bioassay, in which male and female rats (Fischer 344/N) and mice (B6C3F1 hybrid) are exposed to a single chemical at three levels and compared to untreated controls, in groups of fifty animals (Interview S84; see also NTP 2002).

Despite toxicology's many successes, these techniques have shaped also the challenges and lacunae at the center of the consensus critique of contemporary environmental health science. Controlled laboratory environments and highly standardized mice provide toxicologists with a means of ascertaining specific effects of single chemicals: "[T]he environment of the laboratory is carefully constructed so that agency can be ascribed solely to the chemical under study" (Nash 2006: 159). However, outside the laboratory, environments and human bodies are far more variable and complex. As such, scientists' focus on the effects of individual chemicals has contributed to the limitations in our understanding of the effects of chemical mixtures. Likewise, the reliance of laboratory techniques on animal models introduces into risk assessment and regulation the uncertainties associated with cross-species extrapolation.

Despite these limitations, the laboratory ideal embodied in toxicological research has also served as the basis for long-standing critiques of environmental epidemiology, which historically has offered a different approach to understanding the relationships among bodies, the environment, and human health and illness. As we will see, environmental epidemiologists have been at the forefront of efforts to develop molecular measures of the environment and have pioneered the practices of molecular epidemiology. Understanding environmental epidemiology, then, as well as the challenges it has faced, is critical to understanding the emergence of molecular measures of the environment and their complex consequences.

Environmental Epidemiology: From the Outside Looking In?

The dilemmas of environmental epidemiology and the motivations of environmental epidemiologists to develop molecular measures of the environment derive from its position between the field-based approach of sanitary engineering and public health and the laboratory-based methods of toxicology. Environmental epidemiologists trace the history of their field to the Sanitary Movement, with its focus on contaminants in water, food, and housing and its support of public health interventions to improve water supplies, food handling, and general living conditions (Merrill 2008). In the post–World War II period, environmental epidemiologists, like toxicologists, increasingly turned their attention to the human health effects of exposures associated with industrial production. However, in contrast to toxicology's reliance on laboratory testing using animal models, environmental epidemiologists tended to work with data from human populations exposed to chemicals in naturalistic settings (i.e., where people actually live, work, and play) as a means of evaluating the effects of such exposures.

Consequently, in the postwar decades, environmental epidemiologists faced myriad challenges. First, environmental epidemiological research required that the nearly infinite complexity of human lives and environments be rendered into standard questions that could be administered to large numbers of people. Exposure assessment posed an especial challenge, as measurement techniques typically depended either on individuals' recall of complex information or extrapolation from external measurements taken at few points in space and time (Vineis 2004: 945). Environmental epidemiologists refer to exposure assessment as "the Achilles heel" of their research (Perera 1987: 887–888).[8] Exposure

assessment is particularly vexing in environmental epidemiology because most people are exposed to environmental chemicals without their
knowledge[9] and from multiple sources:

> I do pesticide research and in pesticide research it's impossible . . . to
> get any kind of dosimeter unless you're using a biomarker. People just
> don't know what they're exposed to; they have no idea. They may know
> whether or not they use pesticides but they have no idea what com-
> pounds they might be exposed to. And there's a lot of exposure that's
> involuntary and they just don't know it at all. So, if you're trying to do
> epidemiology of environmental pesticide exposure and you're not us-
> ing biomarkers, you're going to get terrible exposure misclassifications
> (Interview S05).

As a consequence, survey and questionnaire methods are often insufficient:

> It's very, very hard to determine what environmental exposures are by
> questionnaire, because most people just don't know what particular
> compound they've been exposed to (Interview S05).

Using measures of the ambient environment likewise is problematic because it requires the assumption that the levels of a contaminant in the
air, water, or soil measured at a few points in time will correspond to its
levels inside the human body (Vineis 2004). As a consequence, as one
regulatory scientist put it, "epidemiology is a sitting duck for uncertainty campaigns" (Michaels 2008: 61).

Further, early environmental epidemiology was quite limited in its
ability to measure specific outcomes of exposure:

> When you think of the early environmental epidemiology studies . . .
> they were really mortality studies. [These] mortality studies maybe had
> monitoring stations during the London fog or in northern Pennsylvania,
> where they have some idea of the magnitude of total particulates from
> some area stations, and have mortality as the outcome (Interview S06).

Whereas environmental epidemiologists studied exposure at the level of
the population, the dominant paradigm for postwar epidemiology in the
United States focused primarily on individual risk factors for chronic diseases (Susser & Susser 1996a, 1996b; see also Brown 2007). The challenges

of measuring environmental exposures and their effects meant that, although environmental epidemiologists might be able to identify large populations at risk (e.g., by virtue of massive environmental exposures), they faced tremendous difficulties in identifying *subpopulations* or *individuals* at risk. As a consequence of these perceived limitations, environmental epidemiology existed at the margins of epidemiology.[10] Put differently, because the laboratory paradigm provided the ideal against which any practice of producing knowledge about the body, the environment, health, and illness was compared, "environmental epidemiology was repeatedly criticized as a kind of second rate field science, fatally hampered by the inability of investigators to control the complex social and environmental realities encountered outside the walls of the laboratory . . . " (Nash 2006: 201).

Thus, in the waning decades of the twentieth century, the field of environmental epidemiology was in an extremely vulnerable position. Many environmental epidemiologists identified strongly with the legacy of the Sanitation Movement, with its field-based methods and focus on controlling the environment as a means of protecting public health. However, they recognized that their divergence from the biomedical model (with its roots in the laboratory) and the risk factor paradigm of post–World War II epidemiology (with its focus on modifiable individual risk factors) undermined the status of the knowledge they produced. Further, because of the contentiousness of the environmental health arena, their work frequently met with overt challenges, not only from other scientists, but from regulated industries and from exposed individuals and communities seeking legal redress for what they contend are environmentally associated illnesses. In legal and regulatory battles, environmental epidemiology was denigrated particularly in comparisons to molecular biology, which scientists touted for offering greater specificity in identifying mechanisms through which chemicals have effects. As noted in Chapter 1, beginning in the 1980s, the National Institute of Environmental Health Sciences (NIEHS) and the National Toxicology Program (NTP) came under significant pressure to fund and conduct research on the molecular mechanisms through which environmental exposures cause adverse health outcomes. And, indeed, in the 1980s, environmental epidemiologists turned to the tools of molecular biology as a means of transforming and strengthening their field.

MOLECULARIZING ENVIRONMENTAL EPIDEMIOLOGY

In 1982, environmental epidemiologist Frederica Perera and her advisor, I. Bernard Weinstein,[11] published the paper that environmental health scientists now point to as the launch of contemporary molecular epidemiology (Perera & Weinstein 1982). In this paper and in subsequent publications, Perera and Weinstein argued that molecular biological techniques could provide important tools for environmental epidemiologists.

Their argument was made up of several interrelated claims. First, Perera and Weinstein asserted that existing epidemiologic approaches were insufficient for detecting and evaluating environmental hazards and their role in human cancer causation. They observed particularly that "the very advantage of epidemiological methods, that they study 'real life' complex human situations, leaves them open to numerous confounding variables" (1982: 583). They thereby acknowledged and endorsed the toxicological critique of environmental epidemiological research. However, at the same time, they pointed to the limitations of animal models in assessing the magnitude of risk posed by a chemical to human populations; that is, they argued that toxicological research was not the answer to the challenges facing environmental epidemiology. Rather, they argued that molecular biological tools offered a means of transcending the limitations of *both* approaches to environmental health research and called for studies that "combine the power of epidemiological techniques with those of recently developed biochemical and molecular methods" (1982: 593). Indeed, an early review described molecular epidemiology as fueled by both the "realization among epidemiologists that substantive advances in our understanding of disease etiology were unlikely to be obtained from better questionnaires" and the realization of "laboratory scientists . . . that humans are not always comparable with inbred strains of rodents" (Ambrosone & Kadlubar 1997: 912).

In support of their argument, Perera and Weinstein identified four types of molecular biomarkers that could be used to improve the practice of environmental epidemiologic research.[12] (1) *Molecular biomarkers of internal dose* indicate the actual level of a compound within the body and/or specific tissues and compartments. (2) *Molecular biomarkers of biologically effective dose* indicate the amount of a compound that has reacted with specific cellular macromolecules. (3) *Molecular biomarkers of effect* identify early biological effects (or response) resulting from exposure. (4) *Molecular biomarkers of susceptibility* are used to identify individual and population differences in susceptibility to adverse outcomes following environmental exposures (Perera & Weinstein 1982). Thus, they asserted, molecular biomarkers would enable epidemiologists to transcend the long-standing methodological challenges of both the field (e.g., confounding) and the laboratory (e.g., extrapolation from animal models) for characterizing the relationships between human bodies, their environments, and human health and illness (Perera & Weinstein 1982: 581–584). As a proof of principle, Perera and Weinstein reported on an assay that allowed them to demonstrate that a known carcinogen (benzo(a)pyrene) had bonded to human DNA; such "carcinogen-DNA adducts" (Figure 3) had the advantage of both proving exposure to a specific chemical and implicating it in a molecular mechanism of cancer causation (i.e., the disruption of DNA replication). Highlighting the centrality of molecular techniques to this new approach to research, Perera and Weinstein called it *molecular epidemiology*. [13]

Molecular epidemiology appealed especially to environmental health scientists who wanted to use laboratory methods to ascertain the health effects of environmental hazards in human subjects, rather than animal models. As a now prominent molecular epidemiologist recounted:

> What I was interested in is molecular mutagenesis—the basic mechanisms of molecular mutagenesis. . . . I had been working on bacterial models of mechanisms. . . . In the 1980s, I switched to studying genetic variations in humans. This is when molecular epidemiology was just getting started. The techniques were being developed and I wanted to get into human studies (Interview S26).[14]

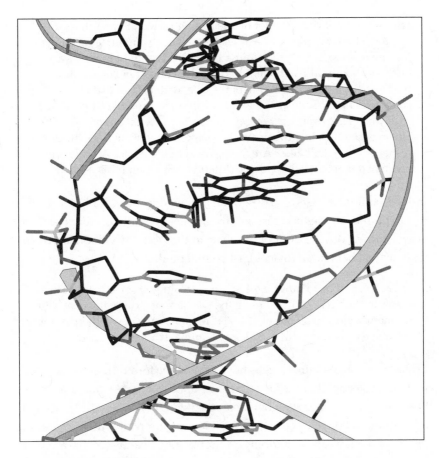

Figure 3. A PAH-DNA adduct.
Source: Created from PDB 1JDG.

Similarly, the potential to do environmental health research using human samples and data attracted the attention and engagement of toxicologists. As this toxicologist commented, he was compelled by the possibility of using molecular biomarkers as a way to transcend the limitations of extrapolating from animal to human models in assessing the risk of environmental chemicals:

> By the end of the 1980's, I had become very disenchanted with animal experiments. . . . I don't really think many of the animal cancer tests are

relevant. I think you get a lot of misleading information with regard to true risk for people. . . . I was challenged at a committee meeting in the late 80's . . . 'what's the alternative?' And I thought that was a good question. So my research went into the direction of biological markers in the late 80's and the beginning of the 90's, with *the idea that we could study people with the latest microbiology and we'd be able to learn a lot more than we could from rats and mice with regard to risk.* So . . . what are people actually exposed to? How much are they exposed to? What does the dose response curve look like? Are there susceptible people? All this could be much better answered in people (Interview S15, emphasis added).

Indeed, some scientists also described organization-wide shifts from animal to human studies as a result of the application of molecular biomarkers. Gesturing out the door of his office to the laboratory doors lining the hallway just beyond, a toxicologist commented:

It has allowed us to move a lot of our toxicology from animals into humans. In the division that I'm in, the Division of Occupational and Environmental Health, all of our studies are in humans now, whereas ten or fifteen years ago we still used a lot of animal studies (Interview S14).

Environmental epidemiologists have been at the forefront of the development of molecular biomarkers and their applications. As one university-based molecular epidemiologist commented, "this is how it [molecular epidemiology] developed . . . the people who got really interested in using these biomarkers were doing environmental health sciences research, looking at effects of environmental exposures . . . " (Interview S05). Contemporary molecular epidemiology combines environmental epidemiologists' focus on ascertaining the effects of the environment on human health and illness with the laboratory-based tools of molecular biology (Interview S04). As I will describe, these applications rest on the capacity of molecular biomarker techniques to give environmental epidemiologists access to the *milieu interieur* of human bodies.

Taking a Look Inside

For environmental epidemiologists, the greatest shift made possible by molecular biomarkers comes from their promise to open up the *milieu interieur* of the human body and render visible, at the molecular level, the chain of events leading from an environmental exposure to an adverse health outcome. Molecular epidemiologists assert that biomarker techniques thereby not only allow them to identify individual and subpopulation risk factors—the paradigmatic focus of postwar epidemiology—but also to address the primary limitation of the risk factor approach. In other words, molecular epidemiologists contend that, in contrast to risk factor epidemiology, which produces "risk ratios that relate exposure to outcome *with no elaboration of intervening pathways*" (Susser & Susser 1996a: 672, emphasis added), biomarkers enable them to elaborate precisely those pathways: "Previously epidemiology mostly was just looking at some kind of exposure determinant and disease; that was it. So that's what the change to molecular epidemiology is about" (Interview S06). Molecular epidemiologists allow that a focus on pathways inside the body already had begun at the time that molecular biomarkers became popular tools in epidemiologic research. [15] These earlier approaches, which were based in biochemistry, allowed environmental epidemiologists to document the presence of a chemical inside the human body. In contrast, molecular biomarkers offer the possibility of not only measuring the presence of a chemical, but also its effects, such as DNA adducts, chromosomal alterations, and somatic mutations (Interview S06). As I will describe, molecular epidemiologists assert that by changing how environmental exposures and their effects are measured, molecular biomarkers provide new opportunities for disease prevention.

Molecular epidemiologists sought first and foremost to improve exposure assessment. According to one researcher, in the early days of molecular epidemiology, "the primary goal was measuring exposure itself" (Interview S26). Molecular epidemiologists point to their desire for more robust and specific exposure assessment as a primary motivation for taking up molecular biomarker techniques:

> We started doing molecular epidemiology because the traditional exposure assessment was not good enough. So, if I wanted to figure out how lead affects neurobehavioral function in adults . . . you would have to take a detailed occupational and environmental history to estimate what the person's exposure was, and I don't think that worked very well. The movement towards biomarkers . . . was to improve on our exposure and dose and risk assessment (Interview S11).

Environmental epidemiologists worried especially that inadequacies in their exposure assessment techniques biased their research toward null results:

> I think one of the reasons, and maybe the most important reason, was to improve our exposure and dose assessment. Lots of studies had been done relying on exposure measures that would report no association between the exposure assessment and the health outcome, and many of us were just worried that those techniques were just too error prone, and that would bias you towards a null finding (Interview S20).

The validation of molecular biomarkers often hinges on issues of dose assessment, as well. As this molecular epidemiologist explained: "We're doing both [internal and external measurements]. And I think you need both because you need to relate it [the molecular biomarker] back to what's out there in the end" (Interview S04). Again, the focus is on tracing pathways from the external environment to inside the human body. Whereas historically an exposure in environmental epidemiological research was "something a person can tell you" that provided an "indirect, categorical surrogate for a predictor of disease risk," from "the molecular epidemiologist's view" an exposure is "something (biomarker) measured inside a person" that "relates directly or indirectly to internal dose" (Rappaport 2010).

In addition to providing better means of doing exposure assessment, molecular biomarkers offer epidemiologists the opportunity to examine what happens inside the human body following an environmental exposure:

> The biomarkers are telling you more than you can get through monitoring, and it's telling you something different. It is telling you not only was there exposure, but it is telling you something about how that individual processed, handled the exposure (Interview S04).

Providing information about how individuals "handle" an exposure is the work of molecular biomarkers of *effect* and of *susceptibility*.[16] In practice, these are complementary tools that are often used in tandem: "[A] lot of people are doing . . . work using biomarkers both of effect and susceptibility and looking at disease modulation" (Interview S04). For example, molecular epidemiologic research suggests that DNA adducts may serve as "an integrated marker of exposure *and* of the individual ability to metabolize carcinogens and repair DNA damage" (Vineis & Perera 2000: 325, emphasis added). Molecular epidemiologists believe that such measures could fundamentally transform the definition of disease phenotypes:

> [The] technologies that are developing are all lending themselves for quantitative measures. We're going to start to define cases [people who are ill] as "you've got one hundred thousand deformed proteins," as opposed to . . . "you have emphysema" (Interview S20).

Molecular epidemiologists frame both kinds of biomarkers as important mechanisms for intervening in environmentally associated disease processes, insofar as they allow for the identification of people at increased risk of illness following an environmental exposure.

MOLECULAR BIOMARKERS IN DISEASE PREVENTION

Molecular epidemiologists articulate a strong shared commitment to disease prevention and public health: "[T]he goal of such research is practical: to apply relevant and valid biomarkers and to incorporate the resulting information into public health actions" (Christiani 1996: 921; see also Hemminki et al. 1996; Perera 1997, 2000). In a presentation to the Molecular Epidemiology Group at the annual meeting of the American Association for Cancer Research (AACR) in 2002, Perera expressed concern that "we don't spend enough time translating our results" and challenged her colleagues to "lay out contexts and frameworks and their importance to prevention." As this discussion unfolded, there was broad agreement among the molecular epidemiologists present that "the goal of molecular cancer epidemiology is to develop early warning systems to prevent cancer onset" (Field Notes, AACR 2002). Nonetheless, molecular epidemiologists vary in their visions of how biomarkers can inform prevention. Some focus on developing clinical interventions to interrupt the disease processes initiated by environmental exposures. Others hope that biomarkers that can be used to determine whether a contaminant in the environment has entered and found "molecular targets" inside a human body will motivate public policy interventions.

Although molecular epidemiologists state clearly that "we are not at the point where we can say to an individual we have measured this marker, that marker . . . therefore your risk is x" (Interview S04), they assert that the identification of disease precursors eventually will increase the period of time during which the risks of disease can be identified, prevented, and/or managed. For example, molecular epidemiologists highlight the possibility that molecular biomarkers may allow scientists to better map, understand, and intervene in the *latency period*, that is, the time following an exposure but prior to onset of any clinical symptoms of disease.[17] Prior to molecular epidemiology, latency was incorporated in environmental epidemiological study designs as a part of efforts to ascertain *when* an exposure occurred. For example, if one were was to investigate the relationship between an environmental chemical and a form of cancer suspected to have a ten-year latency period, one would ask individuals with that cancer about exposures approximately ten years prior to being diagnosed. However, molecular biomarkers of effect give epidemiologists something to measure and to monitor *during* the latency period between the occurrence of an exposure and its suspected effects:

> . . . one area that I think is becoming really well-developed is a better understanding of the idea of latency. Because, you see, latency is a complete artifact of epidemiology. It turns out that latency doesn't really exist. What they teach you in epidemiology is that you have to really figure in five or ten years of latency for solid tumors. . . . But it's not like nothing happened in those five or ten years (Interview S07).

As such, molecular epidemiologists suggest that by identifying the changes that occur during the latency period, it is may be possible to intervene in the disease process and prevent the manifestation of symptomatic disease:

> . . . rather than just looking at exposure to disease relationships, there is now [a way to look at] exposure and intermediate changes in perfectly healthy people that would perhaps go away if the exposure stopped, and then [disease] would not ever be manifested . . . (Interview S20).

Molecular epidemiologists propose that such "intermediate changes" could serve as new diagnostic categories: "We have used phenotype forever to diagnose disease. Now what we're doing is actually looking at that phenotype at the molecular level" (Interview S20). These molecularized models of disease replace step function models of health and illness with one based on continuous gradients of quantifiable markers of disease. A step function model, as described by this molecular epidemiologist, would tell you: "So you're healthy, now you have hypertension, now you have advanced cardiovascular disease, now you have congestive heart failure, now you're dead" (Interview S21). In contrast, a continuous model measures the accumulation of molecular biomarkers and their associated *risks* over the life course. Therefore, from a molecular epidemiologic perspective, one may not be merely healthy or ill; rather, as this epidemiologist described: "What we would do is . . . use biomarkers as . . . measures of disease accumulation . . . *You would be dealing with somebody in a variety of gradations of disease*" (Interview S21, emphasis mine).

Molecular epidemiologists have used biomarkers also to evaluate "individually designed preventions," including eliminating the environmental exposure or providing chemoprevention or dietary supplements to persons identified as at risk. Much of the molecular epidemiological research on the effect of interventions has been done with people who use tobacco products; for example, researchers have studied the effects of smoking cessation and vitamin supplements by measuring levels of adducts associated with tobacco smoke (Garcia-Closas et al. 1997; for a review, see Vineis & Perera 2000). This model assumes an exposure that is subject to some measure of individual control. However, molecular epidemiologists suggest that it would apply also to situations in which the exposure cannot be altered:

> So if you have an individual who is in the workplace and is exposed to an agent in the workplace that could be very toxic, if it's metabolized and converted to a more toxic metabolite, then you might intervene with another agent that would inhibit that enzyme. *That's frequently done in clinical medicine* (Interview S20, emphasis added).

This more biomedical approach to environmental health has been criticized from both within and outside the field. Epidemiologists have

expressed concern especially that in its pursuit of the molecular mechanisms of disease etiology, molecular epidemiology will "shift . . . [the]
focus from the population to the individual" (Ambrosone & Kadlubar
1997: 912–913). Further, as will be detailed in Chapter 6, environmental
health and justice activists observe that molecular epidemiology's focus
on identifying changes caused by environmental exposures may prevent
disease, but only after the fact of harmful exposures. It is unquestionable
that developing post-exposure individual-level clinical interventions is
the focus of some molecular epidemiologists: "What drives my basic science in terms of developing these biomarkers is to really use them as tools
in preventive interventions, which have to be individually based. . . .
In other words, if an individual is exposed, we need to know that exposure, so then we can intervene and drive the effective consequences of
that exposure down" (Interview S21).

However, other molecular epidemiologists are quick to point out
that the identification of biomarkers of effect might serve as a rationale
for policy interventions to remove or limit ongoing environmental exposures (Interview S06); for example, if "data show that we have had
disproportionately high exposure in the community and we need to do
something about it" (Interview S04). Molecular measurements of the environment have met with challenges, however, in community settings.
Molecular epidemiologists are emphatic that they intend their research
to support exposed communities, to "bring them the leverage they need
to effect change" (Interview S04). However, as I describe in the following pages, the case of Midway Village highlights the challenges of using
internal, molecular measures of the environment in community-based
environmental health controversies.

POLLUTION INSIDE AND OUT: MIDWAY
VILLAGE, CALIFORNIA

"Gene Defects for Neighbors of Toxic Site" declared the *San Francisco
Chronicle* headline on January 19, 2000, "Study Finds Aberrations in Chromosomes Among Daly City Project Residents." The study announced in

the headline was an analysis of blood samples from 58 residents of Midway Village, a public housing project in Daly City, California. According to the report of the private medical clinic that conducted the study at the request of Midway Village residents,[18] 32 of 34 children (ages 18 and younger) and 19 of 24 adults had "chromosome aberrations and irregularities" (Pence 2000b). This analysis followed more than a decade of activism by residents of the Midway Village who allege that chemicals in the soil beneath the housing project are responsible for their many health problems, which include a wide range of conditions, such as cancer, respiratory/breathing problems, infertility, birth defects, learning disabilities, skin problems, neurological disorders, heart abnormalities, digestive disorders, seizures, and death (Lerner 2007).

As early as 1997, local newspaper reporters had made a connection between the concerns of Midway Village residents and the practices of molecular epidemiology. An article in the *San Francisco Examiner* noted that "in recent work Frederica P. Perera . . . and other researchers have found that people exposed to polycyclic aromatic hydrocarbons (PAHs) suffered greater than normal levels of genetic mutations and other chromosome disturbances in blood cells" (Kay 1997a). In fact, Perera's proof of principal experiments for the potential of molecular biomarkers in epidemiological research were studies of how human DNA is affected by benzo(a) pyrene, a PAH that is one of the principal contaminants found in the soil at Midway Village (Perera & Weinstein 1982). The chromosomal analyses of Midway Village residents focused not on DNA adducts, however, but on two different molecular measures of DNA damage associated with carcinogenesis: chromosome aberrations and sister chromatid exchange.

The case of Midway Village offers one of the only available examples of what happens when molecular measures of the environment (i.e., inside the human body) enter into community-based environmental health controversies. Environmental health and justice activists reference Midway Village in their analyses of the potential costs and benefits of molecular techniques from the perspective of communities of color. Thus, although it is impossible to know whether—or to what extent—Midway Village is a harbinger of things to come, we have much to learn from what has happened there.[19] In particular, I will argue that the sequence

of events at Midway Village highlight the obstacles facing molecular epidemiological measures of the environment as a basis for environmental
governance, especially insofar as they conflict with extant regulatory
frameworks that are based on measures of the external environment.

Living on Toxic Ground?

The Midway Village Housing Project consists of 150 units in multifamily
townhomes housing approximately 500 residents. It is located immediately adjacent to the site of a former Pacific Gas and Electric (PG&E) gas
manufacturing plant that closed in 1916. In 1944, in an effort to find a
building site for new Navy housing, the U.S. government used its power
of eminent domain to appropriate 10 acres of the PG&E land, as well as
some adjoining private property. Navy contractors used soil from the
PG&E site to fill in marshland, as part of the construction of the barracks,
which remained under the purview of the federal government until after
the Korean War (Salocks 2006). In 1955, the federal government deeded
Midway Village to San Mateo County for public housing and school construction. The current Midway Village residences were constructed in
1976, on 18 acres that include the site of the former barracks (Figure 4).

Building contractors informed federal housing authorities as early as
1944 that the land on which they proposed to build Navy housing was
contaminated with "much decomposed lampblack and oil refuse mixed
with the mud"; however, neither the Navy nor the county conducted
any soil testing at the site prior to building houses there (Kuz 2006: 18).
In 1980, investigators found contaminated soil at a PG&E service center
next to Midway Village, and four years later, the Environmental Protection Agency placed the service center on the Superfund Program list of
the most contaminated industrial sites in California.[20]

As part of the evaluation of the PG&E service center contamination,
testing was conducted on the neighboring Midway Village site; it revealed high levels of PAHs in the soil. Ten months later, PG&E, along
with county and state officials, held a public meeting to inform Midway
Village residents about the contaminated soil. At the meeting they distributed a fact sheet stating that the chemicals in the soil did not pose a

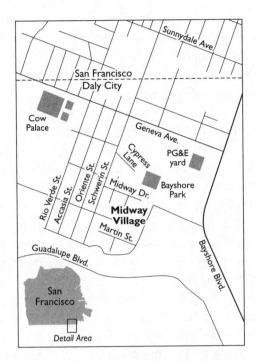

Figure 4. Map of Midway Village, California.
Source: Greenaction for Health and
Environmental Justice.

short-term health risk but that the soil did contain suspected carcinogenic chemicals that posed a long-term risk[21] (Kay 1997a). Then, barely
a month after the public meeting, the state issued an order of "imminent
and substantial endangerment" to PG&E, the U.S. Navy, and the Department of Housing and Urban Development, placing Midway Village on
the state hazardous waste cleanup program.

Both the public meeting and the remediation efforts that followed it
raised alarm among the residents of Midway Village, many of whom had
long been worried about the prevalence of health problems in their community (Kuz 2006). By examining state records, residents learned that
soil in at least three dozen of their front yards and patios, as well as in
public play yards and parts of Bayshore Park and the Bayshore Child

Care Center, was contaminated with 51 chemicals, some at high levels (Kay 1997a). In fact, scientists working for PG&E found benzo(a)pyrene, a PAH classified as a probable human carcinogen, at 150 times normal levels around approximately 36 homes on the PG&E property boundary and at roughly twice normal levels in the child care center area (Kay 1997a). In 1991 and 1993, the state and the housing authority covered open trenches in Midway Village and open soil areas in Bayshore Park. Interventions included removing a top layer of soil and paving over yards and play areas, putting in sidewalks, parking lots, and a slab under the park bleachers, and placing new gravel on the baseball diamond. However, to the frustration of the residents, the soil under the residences at Midway Village was never tested, and consequently no steps were taken to evaluate or ameliorate possible contaminants in it. Moreover, residents reported that their interactions with cleanup workers provided little solace. Speaking to a reporter from the *San Francisco Examiner*, in 1997, Lula Bishop, a resident of Midway Village since 1978, recalled seeing "space-suited workers" digging outside her house one day in 1990 and asking, "Why are you wearing those suits?" "'For the same reason that you should get back in the house and shut that window,' the man yelled back" (Kay 1997a). Advice from health officials—"wear gloves when gardening to avoid skin contact with soil, bathe children multiple times a day if they play outside"—further exacerbated residents' concerns about whether they were living "on toxic ground" (Kuz 2006; Pence 2000b).

The Damaged Gene as a Cultural Icon

Soon after learning about the contamination of their community, Midway Village residents initiated a series of lawsuits, demanding compensation for harms done to them by exposure to toxic chemicals at the Midway Village Housing Complex; some suits asked also for relocation and associated expenses. A class action lawsuit against the federal government, in which 250 residents charged the government with endangering their health and asked for $1.25 million in compensation, was filed in 1993. It was dismissed on the grounds of federal immunity; in other word, the government does not permit itself to be sued in these kinds of cases (Lerner 2007). Residents also sued the San Mateo Housing Authority and PG&E for failing to protect their health. Suits filed against PG&E and the San Mateo Housing Authority were dismissed by trial judges who found that Midway Village residents and former residents had failed to link the chemical exposure to their individual illnesses[22] (Kay 1997b), a common challenge in toxic tort cases (Jasanoff 1995: 119).[23]

The chromosomal analysis undertaken at the request of Midway Village residents must be understood against the backdrop of these court rulings. Specifically, the residents sought DNA data as a means of linking the PAH contamination in the soil at Midway Village to their many ailments (Pence, 2000a). Although the analyses undertaken at the request of Midway Village residents did not ascertain the presence of environmental chemicals inside their bodies, they were meant to establish chromosomal damage as the *mechanism* through which chemicals in the environment had harmed their health.

The announcement that "most residents tested at a San Mateo County housing project built on contaminated soil show an 'abnormal' number of genetic defects . . . " (Pence 2000a) provoked immediate actions from state and county politicians, contrasting sharply with the lassitude of their previous responses. The day after the *San Francisco Chronicle* broke the news of the report, Assemblyman Kevin Shelley (D–San Francisco) announced that his office was requesting an immediate investigation by the California Environmental Protection Agency (Cal/EPA) and had begun exploring options for relocating Midway Village residents[24] (Pence 2000e). Within a week's time, county officials had asked the Department of Housing and Urban Development for emergency funding to permanently relocate tenants of the housing project (Pence 2000c). State lawmakers also met with residents and federal and state toxics regulators to outline a strategy for a health study of Midway Village; during this meeting, state toxics regulators committed to testing 250 soil samples in 100 locations throughout the site and monitoring the air inside residents' homes (Pence 2000b). Meanwhile, lawyers agreed to represent a group of 400 Midway Village residents in new suits that incorporated the chromosomal test results as evidence of environmental harms. One of the lawyers representing the Midway Village residents indicated that he anticipated "getting everyone tested (for gene abnormalities)" as part of preparation for filing the lawsuit (Pence 2000d). Initially, the (damaged) gene worked as a powerful cultural and political icon (Nelkin & Lindee 2004).

Challenging Chromosomes

Despite the rapid response of state and local politicians, the meaning of the chromosomal analysis was contested as soon as it was made public. Scientific assessment of the report of chromosomal damage among Midway Village residents ranged from cautious to critical. Dr. John Wiencke, a molecular epidemiologist at the University of California, San Francisco (UCSF), commented to the *San Francisco Chronicle* that recent scientific studies had indicated that people who have more chromosome aberrations are more prone to some cancers, but he made no comment on the chromosomal analysis itself. Dr. Gina Solomon, a senior scientist at the Natural Resources Defense Council and an assistant clinical professor of medicine at UCSF, asserted, "This is not something that can be ignored. . . . At the very least, it requires investigating more about these people's environment." However, Solomon and others commented also that the report did *not* prove a link between environmental exposures and residents' illnesses (Pence 2000a).

At the request of the Midway Village residents, scientists at the Agency for Toxic Substance and Disease Registry (ATSDR) reviewed the analyses and found them to be "seriously flawed." One critique centered on the absence of any indication as to what constituted normal, above normal, or abnormal levels of chromosomal abnormalities. Likewise, the ATSDR criticized the report for not making an effort to take into account the "normal variability in the population." In summary, the ATSDR review found "the DNA data are inadequate to access current levels of exposure to PAHs at the site" and cannot "predict adverse health effects for individuals living at Midway Village." Additionally, the ATSDR stated that there exists no reliable test that *could* conclusively link PAHs with the residents' many ailments (quoted in Lerner 2007: 15).

The response of state regulatory agencies posed what proved to be an even more critical set of challenges. In February 2001, state toxics regulators announced the results of the soil testing that they had committed to doing following the report of the chromosomal study (Pence 2000c). This analysis found that "chemical levels detected do not represent a serious potential public threat to residents" (Pence 2001b) and did not exceed EPA screening goals,[25] severely undermining the claim that toxic chemicals in the soil are the cause of chromosomal anomalies and illness among Midway Village residents. In 2001, San Mateo County Board of Supervisors President Mike Nevin said he was satisfied that Midway Village was safe. At that time, he instructed the county's Housing Authority to begin filling two dozen vacant apartments in the project (Pence 2001a). Officials from the State Department of Toxic Substances Control held a meeting at Midway Village, at which they informed the tenants that they had concluded that no one needed to be relocated from Midway Village.

A *San Francisco Chronicle* editorial in January of 2000 asserted that "When the soil is abnormally toxic and residents who live on it are getting abnormally sick—as is the case at a San Mateo County housing project—it is not hard to conclude that there is likely a connection between the two." However, as we have seen, even when there is clear evidence of environmental pollution, making the connection between toxics and their health effects is a complex and often contentious process. Scientists developed molecular biomarker techniques, in part, as a means of improving measurements of exposures and their effects, with the goal of elucidating these connections. However, in the absence of evidence of a harmful exposure in the ambient environment—e.g., "abnormally toxic" soil—this causal chain became unmoored. Like the illnesses of the residents, the chromosomal abnormalities could not be associated with a causal factor in the ambient environment (i.e., what is measured and governed under the current regulatory framework), which drastically diminished their epistemic and political power.

Back Outside

Following the announcement of the results of the 2001 soil study, Midway Village residents expressed their mistrust of "government tests" and "reports" about the soil at Midway Village, emphasizing rather their decades-long observation of illness in the community: "'Midway Village is contaminated with toxins, regardless of what government tests say,' said Irma Anderson, who has lived in the complex for 20 years. 'I live here. I know something is making my neighbors sick'" (Pence 2001b). Basila de Guzman, another longtime resident, noted the disjuncture between the reports of government agencies and her observation of her neighbor's health. "I'm tired of these reports," she said, "They can put out report after report saying that we're not sick. But we're sick. I can't breathe. My eyes are watering. My friends are dying of cancer. I don't see any reports on that" (Pence 2001b).

In the years following the Cal/EPA soil study, the controversy at Midway Village has centered not on the residents' *milieu interieur,* but on measurements taken of the *external environment,* with scientists and regulators debating the best means of assessing chemical exposures at Midway Village. Some environmental health scientists have suggested that Cal/EPA's measures of the ambient environment are not adequate measures of human exposure. In fact, this critique emerged prior to the start of the soil study conducted by EPA in 2000–2001. In comments to the *San Francisco Chronicle* in June 2000, Dr. Wayne Ott, a Stanford scientist who specializes in exposure analysis, stated: "To measure the soil and then say this has something to do with exposure is scientific nonsense. When they're done with their soil sampling, they will know absolutely nothing about what these people were exposed to" (Pence 2000f). However, his solution to this problem was not molecular. Rather, he recommended rather that EPA officials use "PNA-monitoring boxes," camera-sized devices containing a pump-and-filter system that records exposures to particles and airborne organic compounds that can be worn on the body. The goal of using these devices would be to assess individual exposure levels, which previous studies have found to be up to 60 percent greater than suggested by measurements of indoor or outdoor air (Pence 2000f). Nonetheless, in the years following the chromosomal analysis, individual exposure assessments have not been conducted; rather, sampling, characterization, and remediation of the site have focused on the ambient environment, especially the soil (Salocks 2006).

The remediation of the site also has been controversial. In September 2005, after hearing testimony from residents of Midway Village, the

Cal/EPA Environmental Justice Advisory Committee (CEJAC) recommended that the Secretary of Cal/EPA initiate a review of the remediation actions at the Midway Village. [26] In response, Cal/EPA tasked its Office of Environmental Health Hazard Assessment (OEHHA) with evaluating whether remedial actions at Midway Village were adequate to fully protect the health of residents living at the complex. Cal/EPA also invited the participation of staff members from the Department of Toxic Substance Control (DTSC), the agency that oversaw the remediation of the site, three members of CEJAC, and the community.[27] Additionally, Cal/EPA hired a technical consultant chosen by the Midway Village residents, Dr. Wilma Subra. Based on its review of "more than 30 reports and background documents dealing with contamination at Midway Village,"[28] the OEHHA review concluded that "there is no disputing that potential 'gaps' in characterization of site contaminants have not been investigated as aggressively as they might have been" (Salocks 2006: 7). Further, it recommended additional studies to evaluate potential exposure to PAHs and volatile organic compounds in indoor air. Nonetheless, the report concluded that:

> . . . the nature and extent of contaminants in surface soil have been adequately characterized for the purpose of assessing potential risks to human health. While contaminants still remain in subsurface soil, minimal opportunities for exposure to these contaminants exist. The remedial actions taken by DTSC, together with ongoing institutional controls on land use, are sufficient to prevent significant exposure to contaminants in surface and sub-surface soil. Since potential pathways for exposure have been blocked or are insignificant, potential health risks are insignificant as well. The remedial actions taken at Midway Village appear to be consistent with federal and state guidelines for management of health risks at hazardous waste sites (Salocks 2006: 1).

Again, the scope of the review focused entirely on the assessment and remediation of the external environment. In their comments on the OEHHA review, members of CEJAC and Dr. Subra similarly focused primarily on the assessment and remediation of the external environment.[29]

Only in the context of the CEJAC discussion of community health analyses are the chromosomal analyses of Midway Village residents mentioned at all. The CEJAC review acknowledges the ATSDR's assessment that the chromosomal analyses were not "useful." At the same time, it suggests that the analyses raise "the question [of] why there have been no further efforts to determine if significant health effects are being observed in the community at Midway" (Salocks 2006: 98). Consequently, the CEJAC recommended that:

> A comprehensive and systematic assessment of the health effects experienced by the residents should be undertaken. . . . *Efforts should be made to clarify or to redo the genetic testing . . . if provocative results such as this are not accepted and acted upon, they should at least be responded to in a more conclusive way* (Salocks 2006: 103, emphasis added).

In an initial consultation with OEHHA, public health experts from the California Department of Health Services (DHS) suggested that "such a study would have great limitations, and the chance that it would generate useful results is small" (Salocks 2006: 2).[30]

Since the Toxic Substances Control Act (TSCA) became law in 1976, toxicological testing to assess the potential of a chemical to cause damage to human DNA has been part of registration (regulatory review) for all new chemical compounds (Frickel 2004). Molecular epidemiologists propose that the mechanisms of DNA damage, such as DNA adducts, can be used to identify people experiencing adverse effects from chemical exposures well in advance of their progression to symptomatic disease. However, as highlighted by the case of Midway Village, regulatory agencies set action and remediation targets for the air, water, and soil. As an environmental health scientist familiar with the controversy explained:

> The [regulatory] process is actually defined by legal requirements and has to do with lawyers . . . . Ultimately clean-up is defining a number that is "safe" and then demonstrating that the strategy has gotten near that number. The issue of whether we have a difference in perception in looking at individual exposure or looking at concentrations in the air *does not enter into this process as it is currently done.* So what we see at Midway Village, or what we see at your house, is that you measure concentrations in the water that is flowing in the aquifer, or you measure concentrations in air, and relate them to some sort of goal that is set by a risk assessment process, and then say 'this is safe or this is not safe' (Interview S13).

As I describe in detail in the following chapter, environmental health scientists have begun to work with federal regulatory agencies to identify opportunities for integrating molecular biomarkers into risk assessment and regulation. Meanwhile, California's DTSC remains focused on the soil at Midway Village, rather than on the chromosomes or the health of the residents. In January 2007, it began a five-year review of the Midway Housing Complex cleanup action to determine whether further steps are necessary to clean up the soil (Lerner 2007).

FROM THE ENVIRONMENT IN THE LABORATORY . . . TO THE LABORATORY IN THE ENVIRONMENT?

In years following Perera and Weinstein's (1982) call for a "molecular epidemiology," this approach to studying the relationships among bodies, the environment, and human health and illness has burgeoned, especially in the United States and Europe (Ugolini et al. 2007). Although, as some scientists pointed out, "the epidemiology—the study design and data analysis—is not that new" (Interview S19), using molecular biomarkers to measure the environment and its effects inside the human body has transformed environmental epidemiology:

> There's a big emphasis, especially when you're doing environmental epidemiology now, on the use of biologic markers. . . . Most studies that are being proposed have a biologic component to it, at this point. And, you know, this is a huge area of research and there's certainly a lot of interest and funding for biomarker validation, too (Interview S05).

Molecular epidemiologists are quick to claim that their success is the result of sustained effort:

> . . . We spent a good part of the last ten years trying to educate people about these markers, develop methods, validate the methods in small studies, convince funding agencies to fund validation studies, and gradually there has been an acceptance, in the field, of the use of biomarkers (Interview S11).

Some assert, however, that their successes go beyond "an acceptance": "there's going to be no epidemiology very soon. . . . It is going to be

molecular epidemiology . . . " (Interview S25). Another molecular epidemiologist stated, somewhat more circumspectly:

> I think in a few years, more epidemiological studies will be us-
> ing molecular methods and biomarkers than don't. If you design an
> epi[demiology] study now and you're not at least considering saving
> tissues or samples or buccal swabs or blood or urine or something for
> analysis later, you're probably missing the boat. . . . I think it will become
> the primary approach in the near future (Interview S12).

Molecular epidemiological techniques have been taken up especially in
large longitudinal cohort studies, such as the National Children's Study,
which seek to ascertain how environmental exposures affect health and
development at the population level. [31]

In facilitating the identification of environmental contaminants inside the human body and at the molecular level, molecular biomarker
techniques have provided environmental epidemiologists with new
means of measuring the environment. For molecular epidemiologists,
the environment is represented not only by the specific chemicals that
can be measured in the blood, urine, or other samples collected from
human subjects, but also by their molecular consequences, such as
chemical adducts attached to human DNA. Molecular epidemiologists
use varied techniques, then, for correlating these measurements of the
human *milieu interieur* with measures of the environments in which research subjects actually live and work. Often, molecular epidemiological research combines and/or compares internal and external measures
of the environment. For example, in a study that used levels of DNA
adducts to examine the effects of air pollution on pregnant women and
their children, scientists estimated each woman's exposure to ambient
particulates by taking the average of particulate matter ($PM^{10)}$) measurements reported at the air quality monitoring station closest to her
residence for the year prior to her delivery date (Whyatt et al. 1998).
In this way, molecular biomarker techniques provide environmental
epidemiologists with a way of combining "an approach oriented toward biology and the study of mechanisms, and an approach oriented
to populations and their interactions with the environment" (Parodi,

Neasham, & Vineis 2006: 358). In published commentaries about the future of their field, epidemiologists have suggested that answering questions about the relationships between the environment and human health requires that research focus simultaneously on both the external environment and the *milieu interieur* (Loomis & Wing 1990; Susser 1998; Susser & Susser 1996a, 1996b). In fact, some environmental epidemiologists propose that the ongoing tensions between "the laboratory" and "field work," between identifying "biological mechanisms" and "the study of populations," is "in fact essential for the success of the discipline" (Parodi et al. 2006).

Molecular epidemiology has been especially prominent in epidemiological research on the environmental causes of cancer. As noted by Wild (2010), first-generation molecular biomarkers were "based in the carcinogen model of carcinogenesis" and "tended to focus on a classical mutagen" and its effects (e.g., metabolites, adducts, chromosomal alterations, somatic mutations).[32] Additionally, a molecular epidemiologist commented that with its long latency period, cancer was "calling out for this kind of research and with enormous potential for prevention, given the fact that often decades intervene between first exposure and cancer itself" (Interview S04). At the 2002 meeting of the American Association of Cancer Research, 81% (400/496) of all paper and poster submissions to the Epidemiology Section reported on the results of molecular epidemiologic research (Field Notes, AACR 2002). In the past 25 years, molecular epidemiologists have published studies showing a correlation between external measurements of exposure and biomarkers of early biological response/effect for multiple environmental chemicals, demonstrated that there are overall correlations between DNA or protein adduct levels and environmental exposures (with significant interindividual variation in adduct levels), confirmed that carcinogen-DNA adducts and chromosome aberrations can be used to predict cancer, and identified genetic variants that modulate the risk of cancer in subjects exposed to carcinogens (Vineis & Perera 2007: 1954). In addition to serving as the basis for the development of interventions targeted to people at risk, findings from molecular epidemiological research have been used in the assessment of environmental hazard identification by the International Agency

for Research on Cancer (IARC), thereby potentially contributing to public policy approaches.[33]

Molecular epidemiology also informs current initiatives in exposure
biology. Prominent molecular epidemiologists have called for investment to "empower exposure assessment," noting that "genotyping is in
fact much more accurate than the vast majority of methods used to measure environmental exposures" (Vineis 2004: 945). As noted in Chapter 3,
the NIH's Genes, Environment, and Health Initiative (GEI) has directed
funding to the development of methods of exposure assessment that will
better "capture the individual and dynamic extent of the exposure and
its impact on fundamental biological processes" (Schwartz & Collins
2007: 695). The impact of molecular epidemiological techniques is evident in GEI's Exposure Biology Program, which emphasizes that adequate exposure assessment will need to "record *internal, molecular events*
that signify increased risk of disease from exposures to different forms
of environmental stress, such as patterns of gene or protein expression,
as well as to measure response indicators *such as DNA or protein adducts*
that persist even after the exposure has ended" (Schwartz & Collins 2007:
316, emphasis added). One goal of the Exposure Biology Program is to
use lab-on-a-chip technology (i.e., small-scale sensing devices) that can
be easily carried or even worn by individuals and will allow for immediate and on-site analysis of environmental exposures and their molecular
effects (Smith & Rappaport 2009). Interestingly, the lab-on-a-chip would
bring environmental health research practices back out into lived environments, while maintaining molecular epidemiology's focus inside the
human body and at the molecular level.

Molecular epidemiology has not been without its critics. As noted,
epidemiologists have expressed concern especially that, in its pursuit of
the molecular mechanisms of disease etiology, molecular epidemiology
would shift the focus of the field from the population to the individual
(Ambrosone & Kadlubar 1997: 912–913). As we have seen, molecular biomarkers have the effect of making environmental exposure a trait that is
measured inside the human body. By looking at chemicals—and their
consequences—inside the human body and at the molecular level, the
risks they pose to our health become *individual* traits. This approach thus

comports well with the dominant epidemiological paradigm (Brown 2007), with its emphasis on modifying individual behavior as a public health strategy. It also aligns environmental epidemiology with the biomedical model, opening up the possibility of new clinical interventions for people who have been exposed to harmful substances in the environment. These innovations address two vulnerabilities of environmental epidemiology as a field. However, they also undermine its traditional orientation to informing population-based interventions to protect public health.

To be sure, many molecular epidemiologists intend for their research to serve as a basis for improving environmental risk assessment and regulation. However, the case of Midway Village demonstrates that molecular measures of the environment and its effects inside the human body face limits as a basis for environmental regulation and public policy. Simply put, molecular measures have no place in extant regulatory frameworks that focus on measurements of the ambient environment. However, for nearly a decade, environmental health scientists, regulators, and policy makers have been working to establish a role for the science of gene-environment interaction in the process of environmental risk assessment. The following chapter examines these efforts.

FIVE Making a Molecular Regulatory Science

> We can do all this environmental research, but until we
> translate that into . . . routine testing methods, then we
> really haven't benefited public health . . .
>
> Interview S34

> [We] don't want this, in the end, to come to some loggerhead
> because labor unions are fighting industry and environmen-
> tal groups. We want everybody to buy into the technology
> before we have it, and before anything is out there. Once
> they buy in and they have signed off on it, they can't just
> change their mind because they didn't like the outcome. . . .
> We want to eliminate that conflict and opposition.
>
> Interview S37

The possibility that genomic data could improve environmental risk assessment and regulation constitutes a central rationale for environmental health scientists' research on gene-environment interaction. However,
as we have seen, the formal policies, practices, and organization of the
regulatory agencies shape whether and how molecular measurements
enter into environmental risk assessment and regulation. At the time that
Midway Village residents announced that chromosomal aberrations had
been found in their blood samples, there was no place for such information in Cal/EPA's analysis of environmental health risks at that site.

An earlier version of this analysis appeared as Shostak, S. "The Emergence of Toxicogenomics: A Case Study of Molecularization." *Social Studies of Science* 35(3): 367–403.
Copyright © 2005 SAGE.

Rather, environmental risk assessment and regulation relied on measures of the ambient environment to assess levels of contamination in the air, water, and/or soil and on animal bioassays to define permissible exposure limits.

However, in 2007, even as Cal/EPA was beginning yet another review of its cleanup of the soil at Midway Village, prestigious committees at the National Academy of Sciences (NAS) were recommending that toxicological testing "take advantage of the on-going revolution in biology and biotechnology" (NRC 2007b). Within a year, the Environmental Protection Agency (EPA), National Institute of Environmental Health Sciences (NIEHS), National Toxicology Program (NTP), and National Human Genome Research Institute (NHGRI) had signed a memorandum of understanding instantiating their commitment to "transform environmental health protection" by using high-throughput screening tools to study the molecular pathways that are perturbed by chemical exposures (Collins, Gray, & Bucher 2008; EPA 2008) and molecular biomarkers to track exposures and health outcomes (Firestone et al. 2010: 152).

This chapter examines how new, molecular scientific practices and the knowledge they generate are becoming part of regulatory science. In contrast to research that describes debates and decision making regarding specific policy problems (e.g., Keller 2009), my focus is on efforts to change aspects of the *process* of environmental risk assessment and regulation by incorporating molecular genomic data. As we will see, such efforts face numerous obstacles. As noted in a government committee report on the development and validation of new toxicological tests:

> Regulatory agencies do not readily accept new and revised test
> methods . . . Hurdles that must be overcome are lack of valid methods,
> bias on the part of scientists and managers both inside and outside
> of regulatory agencies, fear of litigation due to purported absence of
> sensitivity of new methods, and the work involved to change guidelines,
> regulations, or statutes (ICCVAM 1997: 45).

As a consequence, as one toxicologist stated starkly, in risk assessment, "much of the methodology we are using for analysis is, for want of a better term, classical. . . . Certainly these methods have become very straightforward and reliable. . . . Whether they are the most sensitive or not? Usually they are not" (Interview S13).

The procedural conservatism of the regulatory agencies must be understood within the context of the politics of environmental regulation "where there are real winners and losers . . . [and] as a consequence, regulatory agencies face organized and hostile interests" (Keller 2009: 141). The processes of rule making and formal procedures within regulatory agencies act as a stable referent for policy makers and stakeholders. Insofar as they reduce uncertainty about what will be accepted by stakeholders and the courts as legitimate policy, established regulatory protocols protect the legitimacy of the regulatory agencies and reduce the likelihood that they will face legal challenges (Keller 2009). Consequently, environmental health scientists recognize that "the agencies are not going to sacrifice and back away from the standard of protection that they currently have" unless they are certain that the new, alternative testing method "provides for at least equivalent protection of human health, or the environment . . . as the currently used methods or approaches" (Interview S34). More broadly, scholars have noted that standards have significant inertia and can be very difficult to change (Bowker & Star 2000: 14).

Environmental health scientists are well aware of these hurdles and have acted strategically to address them.[1] In fact, a central argument of this chapter is that how scientists and policy makers anticipate, encounter, and respond to these challenges has shaped the emergence of new forms of genomic science. I focus particularly on the science of toxicogenomics, which is one of the high-throughput techniques at the center of the proposed transformation of environmental regulation.

Focusing on toxicogenomics offers several analytic advantages. First, toxicogenomics utilizes a specific technology, the microarray, that was not developed originally by or for environmental health scientists. Therefore, examining its uptake by environmental health researchers provides a means of tracing some of the processes and pathways through which genomic technologies have traveled within and across institutions committed to environmental health research and regulation. Second, soon after they began to operate a microarray facility, NIEHS scientists became interested in the potential regulatory applications of microarray technology, and the

NIEHS took an active role in providing funding for intramural and extramural research aimed at preparing toxicogenomics for use in risk assessment. This has included efforts to bring together scientists, bioethicists, lawyers, and policy makers to anticipate and address the requirements of environmental risk assessment at the EPA (e.g., NRC 2007a, 2007b; Sharp, Marchant, & Grodsky 2008). Consequently, in the case of toxicogenomics, I was able both to collect data on what scientists say about how molecular genetic and genomic technologies will transform risk assessment and regulation, as well as to observe some of the strategies they have undertaken to realize their vision of the future. Third, and related, toxicogenomics served as the first focus of what has become an ongoing effort to bring a wide variety of stakeholders into conversation about how to transform environmental health risk assessment and regulation (NRC 2007a). As we have seen, proponents of both environmental genomics and molecular epidemiology seek to simultaneously maintain the relationships between environmental health research and risk assessment and to develop new, biomedical applications. In contrast, proponents of toxicogenomics—and related high-throughput screening technologies—are seeking to "revolutionize" the process of risk assessment and regulation. For the field of the environmental health sciences, this is a different kind of struggle; it is an effort to increase the autonomy of the environmental health sciences by convincing the regulatory agencies that new, molecular forms of research are important to their work. Thus, the case of toxicogenomics provides us with a vista onto how scientists with professional—and personal—commitments to informing public policy try to shape the markets for their research.

Throughout, the analysis is informed by the sociological literature which highlights the importance of both structural and cultural mechanisms of diffusion. As such, I examine the role of social networks and institutional ties, as well as culturally mediated processes, such as learning, emulation, and communication (Simmons, Dobbin, & Garrett 2008; Strang & Soule 1998). This analysis demonstrates that understanding the diffusion of high-throughput sequencing in environmental health science, risk assessment, and regulation requires that we attend both to structural connections and culturally mediated processes of connecting (Strang & Soule 1998: 276).

The chapter proceeds in four parts. The first describes the debut of microarray technology and its early adoptions in both pharmaceutical research and at the National Institutes of Health (NIH). Second, I examine the diffusion of DNA microarrays to the NIEHS and elaborate on the emergence of toxicogenomics. The third section considers how NIEHS scientists have sought to facilitate the adoption of toxicogenomics as a part of environmental risk assessment. Here, I situate these efforts in relation to the procedural conservatism of the regulatory agencies and the formal requirements of the validation of alternative toxicological methods for use in risk assessment and regulation. Fourth, the chapter examines efforts to establish a consensus among diverse and often antagonistic stakeholders about the meaning of genomic information and its appropriate applications in regulatory contexts–activities that have been supported by the consensus critique. Specifically, I demonstrate that by effacing stakeholders' very different substantive political commitments, the consensus critique has facilitated the emergence of new networks and projects that aim to advance the molecularization of environmental regulation.

THE DEBUT AND EARLY DIFFUSION OF CDNA MICROARRAYS

Microarray technology made its scientific debut in 1995, when Pat Brown and his colleagues at Stanford University published a paper in the prestigious journal *Science* entitled "Quantitative Monitoring of Gene Expression Patterns with a Complementary DNA Microarray" (Schena et al. 1995). In this paper, they described a high-capacity system that they built to monitor the expression of many genes in parallel. This system relied on high-speed robotic printing of complementary DNA (cDNA) onto glass slides (chips) that were then used in quantitative expression measurements of the corresponding genes. As the authors reported, this system enabled them to make differential expression measurements of 45 genes from the small flowering plant *Arabidopsis* using simultaneous, two-color hybridization.

Conceptually, microarray technology is similar to two standard laboratory techniques used to study gene expression: the Northern blot and the
Southern blot (Bartosiewicz et al. 2000). As such, scientists were familiar
with the underlying logic of gene expression profiling. However, the scale
of analysis made possible by DNA microarrays was unprecedented. For
example, a Northern blot generally provides information on 10 or 20 or,
more rarely, up to 100 genes at a time. In contrast, the robotized arrayer
designed by Brown and his colleagues allows researchers to "spot" up to
15,000 genes onto one glass slide and to identify gene expression profiles
for each gene simultaneously using confocal microscopy. In essence, a
cDNA microarray enables a researcher to obtain the results of thousands
of Northern blot experiments simultaneously. As such, both the kind
and the volume of data produced by microarray analysis are remarkable
(Rockett & Dix 1999). Scientists working with microarray analysis often
refer to the amount of data they generate as "mountains" or "tsunamis"
or "seas" worth (Field Notes, NIEHS June 2002). A NIEHS postdoctoral
researcher remarked to me: "Before this [research with cDNA microar-
rays] I had never worked on a study with more than 10 data points, but
this one had 30,000" (Field Notes, NIEHS June 2002).

Another advantage of microarray analysis is that it can support quantitative comparison of global gene expression between virtually any two
biological samples: "One can compare, for example, two different tissues, normal versus diseased tissue or untreated versus exposed cells"
(Lobenhofer et al. 2001: 881). Likewise, one can examine gene expression in cells that have been exposed to a chemical as compared to those
that have not (Hamadeh et al. 2002b). Because of these capacities, scientists have hailed microarray technology as a "revolutionary" means of
performing genome wide expression analysis across various biological
models (Lobenhofer et al. 2001).

Making Connections at the National Institutes of Health

In 1996, soon after the debut of microarrays in *Science*, Jeff Trent, then the
scientific director of the NHGRI, established the first microarray facility
at the NIH. According to his colleagues at the NIH, Trent had been "very

astute" in realizing "the power" of this technology and had worked with Pat Brown in developing it (Barrett, Oral History Interview February 2004). Then, with the assistance of Stanford researchers, Trent and his colleagues built their own robot and scanners and began to explore the potential of microarray technology for analyzing gene expression patterns in human cancers (see, for example, DeRisi et al. 1996).

At the time, Trent and J. Carl Barrett, then scientific director of the NIEHS "were working together on some other projects" and in their conversations about their work Trent noted that microarrays were "a really good technology" (Barrett, Oral History Interview February 2004). Barrett believed that "this could really be useful for toxicology" and, given the novelty of the technology and its potential importance to biomedical research, the NHGRI leadership felt that it was important that other Institutes be able to explore microarray research (Interview S60). Consequently, Trent and scientists from NHGRI offered to assist NIEHS in building a microarray facility.

The NHGRI's assistance to the NIEHS was critical because, before the commercialization of the technology, as this molecular biologist recounted, "unless you had an in with someone who knew how to build the instrumentation, you had no way to even start to do anything with it" (Interview S60). A biomedical engineer recalled:

> [When] Pat Brown came out with his paper, there were no commercially available microarray scanners, microarray printers, you had to make your own . . . early on in the microarray days making your own equipment was the status quo, your only option (Interview S40).

In 1997, Cynthia Afshari, the Group Leader in Dr. Barrett's laboratory, went to NHGRI to learn how to work with microarray technology. She also began to consult extensively with the NIH engineers who were building a robotized arrayer and a scanner for the NIEHS. Building the machinery and obtaining all the materials NIEHS researchers would need to run experiments took about a year. In 1998, with the continued support of NHGRI, the NIEHS began to operate its own microarray machine. The initial focus of microarray research at NIEHS reflected its collaborative origins, as NIEHS scientists collaborated with NHGRI researchers in investigating the uses of microarrays for research on carcinogenesis.

However, as with other genomics initiatives at the NIEHS, the imperative to find "our niche" soon led to the development of toxicologically focused applications.

INSTITUTIONALIZING MICROARRAYS AT THE NATIONAL INSTITUTE OF ENVIRONMENTAL HEALTH SCIENCES

Eager to investigate the utility of microarray technology for the Institute's intramural research program, scientists working with the new microarray machinery at NIEHS began a concerted effort to engage interested intramural scientists and to explore how the technology could be applied to their varied research projects:

> We had a lot of conversations with different people . . . to see what would they do if they had this type of technology. We had a lot of things that we wanted to do with it as far as answering basic research questions, addressing things, helping clone genes, and different kinds of small projects that we would use it for (Interview S60).

From the outset, the leaders of the microarray initiative were focused on developing the applications of microarrays as a tool that could serve the extant research agendas of scientists at the NIEHS:

> We didn't start initially as this big National Center for Toxicogenomics running out of NIEHS. . . . We were just starting based on [the question] what does a single, individual PI [principal investigator] want to do to enhance their research? (Interview S60).

At the same time, researchers at the NIEHS microarray facility also began to think about how microarray technology and gene expression profiles could be applied to serve the specific mission of the NIEHS. As a scientist involved in these initiatives recounted: "This is the National Institute of Environmental Health Sciences. So, *we were looking for our niche*. We didn't need or want to compete with Pat Brown or Jeff Trent" (Interview S32, emphasis added). Toxicology and environmental health research define the jurisdiction of the NIEHS, as he further describes: "What is distinctive here is the National Toxicology Program, the focus on environmental insults, the practice of toxicology" (Interview S32). Conscious of such jurisdictional issues, the researchers working in the NIEHS Microarray Center sought to define a research agenda for exploring applications of gene expression profiling specific to toxicology.

The overlapping concerns of the fields of pharmacology and toxicology and the early applications of microarray technologies in pharmaceutical research provided a jumping-off point for NIEHS researchers interested in developing microarrays as a tool for research in toxicology. As we saw in Chapter 3, the metabolism and detoxification of pharmaceuticals and environmental chemicals involve similar (and sometimes identical) processes. Consequently, a Stanford microarray analysis of the responses of sixty cancer cell lines (the "NCI-60") to pharmaceutical agents suggested that microarrays might similarly be used to investigate how cells respond to environmental chemicals. As a genomics researcher who worked in the Brown laboratory later recounted:

> One of the first experiments that we did was what we call the NCI-60 study, which was to do gene expression profiling on a set of sixty cell lines. These sixty cell lines were tested versus . . . sixty thousand different chemical compounds. So there was a huge database of drug sensitivity on these cell lines. And we then did expression profiling to look for correlations between gene expression patterns and drug sensitivity. *So from the start a toxicology study was actually the first study that we did and published* (Interview S46, emphasis added).

Of particular import to the project of developing a toxicology-specific microarray research agenda, the results of that study indicated that gene expression profiling could facilitate comparisons of how different tissues responded to drugs. Therefore, it stood to reason that gene expression profiling could facilitate comparisons of how different tissues responded to environmental chemicals.

In addition to providing a conceptual rationale for using gene expression profiling in toxicology, environmental health scientists pointed to the adoption of microarrays in pharmaceutical research as a warrant for their development in environmental health research. Biotech and pharmaceutical companies were early adopters of microarrays. Pharmaceutical companies were particularly eager to use microarrays to prescreen drug candidates, thereby potentially reducing the cost of drug development. Writing in *Toxicological Sciences* in 2000, scientists from AstraZeneca observed that "a major part of the developmental cost of every successful new pharmaceutical or agrochemical product is the recovery costs of compounds that have failed in development, due to potential or observed toxicity" (Pennie et al. 2000: 278). Most expensive to pharmaceutical companies are the drugs that fail late in the development process, during clinical trials. In addition, as noted in a *New York Times* article on microarrays and product testing, in the late 1990s "several drugs that were already on the market were removed because they caused harm" (Pollack 2000). Pharmaceutical researchers saw microarrays as one way of meeting the imperative of the industry that dangerous compounds "fail fast, fail cheap" (Pollack 2000). As a toxicologist observed, pharmaceutical companies "had huge amounts of money which enabled them to move quickly in that regard . . . in a very practical way because they have practical goals . . . driven by marketing decisions" (Interview S35).

In contrast, environmental health scientists contended, because there was no profit motive to drive technology development in their field, without NIEHS's investment in microarray research, environmental risk assessment would become outdated and obsolete: "[I]n the environment, it's more for the public good, without the big bucks waiting at the end of the line . . . [so] the environmental health sciences are lagging behind the pharmacological sciences pretty dramatically" (Interview S14). A molecular epidemiologist similarly pointed to the absence of private sector institutions and investment as a liability for the development of environmental health research by noting that ". . . in the San Francisco area there are obviously an enormous number of biotechnology firms. And how many equivalent environmental technology firms are there? Probably . . . none. And that to me always has been the Achilles heel . . ." (Interview S20). The claim being made in such statements is that, in the absence of market incentives, government funding for research plays a critical role in ensuring that the best science is available to support the public good, in this case, the toxicological tests, risk assessment, and regulatory process mandated to protect public health.

Together, these arguments were deployed to support the development of a set of practices that NIEHS researchers called toxicogenomics: "[W]e started to think, could we really use this to advance how we conduct toxicology tests today? That's where the concepts and the ideas of toxicogenomics started to be developed" (Interview S27). In 1999, a team of NIEHS and NCI scientists published the first paper using the term *toxicogenomics* in the journal *Molecular Carcinogenesis* (Nuwaysir et al. 1999). The authors defined toxicogenomics broadly as "a new scientific subdiscipline derived from a combination of the fields of toxicology and genomics" (Nuwaysir et al. 1999: 153). Although some of the authors of the paper recount that a sense of "playing around" with words led to the coining of the term, they also were very aware of wanting to highlight the environmental and toxicological foci unique to their research:

> We started thinking about, well what are our applications? What's relevant to the institute? What should we call this? . . . We weren't doing sort of classic toxicology and we wanted to get across genomics technologies. At the time pharmacogenomics was already being used . . . and we felt like that didn't really describe what we were doing, because pharmacogenomics, while some of it does focus on toxicology, is more focused on drug targets and efficacy kinds of issues. So we felt like ours was really different. . . . We weren't doing sort of classic toxicology and we wanted to get across genomics technologies (Interview S30).

Having a specific term and a distinctive research agenda was important not only for disseminating information about the applications of microarrays to toxicological practice, but also for gaining access to the institutional and financial resources needed by the NIEHS Microarray Center: "We were trying to justify a program and build a program . . . and so [the question was] 'what do we call it?'" (Interview S30). The term *toxicogenomics* met all these needs. By referring specifically to toxicology, it highlighted the unique institutional focus of the NIEHS, while the inclusion of *-omics* made clear that this was a molecularized science. Moreover, itself a neologism, *toxicogenomics* signaled that this was a new set of research practices and would require new resources.

The work of developing and applying microarrays to toxicological research soon became a primary research focus for the scientists working at the NIEHS microarray facility. Central to these initial efforts was NIEHS scientists' development of a custom cDNA microarray chip, called a *ToxChip*, that contained copies of approximately 2,000 human genes with which toxicologists could begin to assess the gene expression profiles of known toxicants. Soon after, the researchers created a chip called the *Human ToxChip*, which contained 12,000 genes, allowing for the evaluation of a substantially greater number of gene expression changes in response to chemicals. ToxChips were especially important to the NIEHS researchers because they concretized a distinctive *toxicological* application of microarray research. Using ToxChips, researchers could investigate the gene expression profiles created by exposures to environmental toxicants. Such specific gene expression profiles could make contributions in research on mechanisms and pathways of toxic response, biomarkers of exposure and effect, and the classification of unknown or novel chemical compounds.

Based on early research with the ToxChips, the leadership of the NIEHS became "bullish" (Field Notes, NIEHS 2002) about the potential of such chips in toxicology research and especially "to revolutionize the screening of chemicals" (NIEHS 2000a). In February 2000, the NIEHS microarray facility was elevated from a collaborative unit within Carl Barrett's laboratory to a center, that is, a core structure at the NIEHS. As a center, the microarray initiative was given its own directors, faculty, staff, and resources to continue the adaptation of microarrays as tools for toxicological purposes.

The NIEHS Microarray Center was an important organizational space for the development of toxicogenomics, especially because it provided scientists with an opportunity to form interdisciplinary collaborations and develop new skills. To do its work, the Center assembled a multidisciplinary team of twelve scientists, representing the wide variety of practices implicated in toxicogenomics:

> We realized early on that we were going to have to have a really multidisciplinary team to be able to put this together. That we were going to need to have computational biologists, bioinformaticists, computer support people, bioengineers, as well as molecular biologists and toxicologists as part of our team (Interview S60).

Related, bioinformatics is required to "make sense" of microarray data for toxicological research:

> Genomics is a paradigm shift [for toxicology] because it is big science. It generates thousands of data points. So, you are dependent on bioinformatics and algorithms to help you mine the data. . . . The information is stored in the data. But we need tools to help us see what is there, to visualize the data (Interview S32).

In addition to requiring new collaborative relationships, the vast amounts of data produced by microarray analyses require new skills and practices of biologists and toxicologists. A genomics researcher described the effects of these changes in the following way: "I used to spend all my time at the bench. Now I spend all my time at the computer" (Interview S46). In addition, taking advantage of the potentials of microarrays in hypothesis-generating research requires a different mind-set than the hypothesis-testing model of traditional toxicology.

> [Toxicogenomics] also requires new training and a different mind-set. Because toxicogenomics can be a hypothesis testing or a hypothesis generating tool. This is a paradigm shift for NIEHS, that it can be a discovery tool. I think that it is important that the technology be used both ways—hypothesis testing and generating. It is so exciting to be in a discovery mode . . . to be thinking about different data sets and tools and how we can do discovery. It's really a tremendously exciting time (Interview S32).

With the elaboration of these molecular toxicological practices, the leadership of the NIEHS increased its commitment to "revolutionize" the field of toxicology through the further development of toxicogenomics (NIEHS 2000a).

In December 2000, the NIEHS announced the establishment of the National Center for Toxicogenomics (NCT) (NIEHS 2000b). The press release emphasized the "application of powerful new techniques" with the potential to transform the discipline of toxicology. As a scientist at NIEHS commented on the founding of the NCT: "The primary push behind it was that this technology had the opportunity to revolutionize toxicology research, literally, and completely transform the way that toxicology research was done" (Field Notes, NIEHS July 2002). A senior scientist at the NCT recalled the process leading up to the announcement of the Center as follows:

> With the rapid progress in the genome arena it was becoming obvious that there were some technologies evolving that could have a real profound effect in toxicology, the capacity, used the right way, to actually change the whole field of toxicology over a period of time (Interview S39).

The official overall objective of the NCT was to "promote the evolution of gene and protein expression technologies and their use to understand adverse environmental effects on human health" (NCT 2002: 4). The NCT was to "foster development in this burgeoning field" (NCT 2002: 13) or, in the words of a NCT scientist, to "create the infrastructure needed for the emergence of toxicogenomics" (Field Notes, NIEHS July 2002).

The "infrastructure needed" was defined, in part, by challenges facing the field. For example, toxicogenomics requires that researchers with diverse backgrounds, expertise, and research practices work together. Therefore, the NCT established a collaborative interdisciplinary Tox/ Path Team, consisting of approximately 20 researchers with expertise in the fields of genomics, bioinformatics, toxicology, and pathology, charged with learning each other's languages and practices. As a self-described "old-school" pathologist working at the NCT vividly described the challenge of learning the language of molecular level research:

> For toxicologists and pathologists, the language of genomics is daunting. We don't have expertise at the genomic level. It makes you feel like you are a fish out of water. And with all the jargon and terminology relating to the genome, it's like being in another country, like being in France and not speaking French (Interview S42).

He also commented on the challenges that face researchers who want to work in toxicogenomics but who are unfamiliar with the language and practices of traditional toxicology: "A lot of geneticists work with yeast. They're not aware of the complexities of whole animals—things like diet, circadian rhythms, and disease" (Interview S42). Indeed, in his assessment, the fact that many genomics researchers lack familiarity with the animals and animal models—currently the primary work objects in toxicological testing—threatens the validity of their research:

> Of course they have the same problems. I asked someone at a meeting about a "liver lobe" and he asked if I meant "the first" when I referred to the "left lateral". Another example is that we do all of our work with male rats because of the menstrual cycle. The genomicists at [a university] were working with female rats. They said that they thought that "it would even out". This is not comforting . . . there is no "evening out" and [if you think so] your experiments . . . are going to be misleading (Interview S42).

A toxicologist vividly characterized the differences between expertise of toxicologists with animal models and that of the mathematicians who provide the bioinformatics expertise required for the analysis of gene expression profiles as follows: "These mathematicians don't know a mouse from a Ford Taurus, but they're necessary. We really need a variety of disciplines working together" (Field Notes, NIEHS July 2002).

The differences between genomic analyses and animal bioassays—and efforts to reconcile them—took especial significance in the context of the NCT's mission to establish a role for toxicogenomics in chemical testing, risk assessment, regulation, and policy making. As described in a NCT brochure: "The NCT aims to use and promote toxicogenomics as a means to guide federal agencies and legislators in developing guidelines and laws that regulate the levels of various chemicals in the environment" (NCT 2002: 13). Achieving a molecular revolution in toxicology would require that toxicogenomics and its products (e.g., gene expression profiles) be understandable and useful within a regulatory system built around the results of animal testing (Schmidt 2009). Consequently, translation and standardization emerged as focal activities of the NIEHS.[2]

RELEVANCE, RELIABILITY, AND REVOLUTION IN TOXICOLOGY

At stake in the efforts of environmental health scientists to translate and standardize toxicogenomics is not just the outcome of a specific regulatory controversy, but rather the formal requirements of the process of testing chemicals, assessing their risks to human health and the environment, and regulating their uses. Evaluating alternatives to the existing process of risk assessment and regulation itself has been governed by public policy since 1993, when the NIH Revitalization Act (Public Law 103-43) required NIEHS to establish criteria for the validation of alternative toxicological testing methods and recommend a process to achieve their regulatory acceptance.[3] To meet this mandate, the NIEHS established an ad hoc Interagency Coordinating Committee on the Validation of Alternative Methods (ICCVAM), consisting of representatives from fifteen U.S. federal agencies.[4] Following the recommendations of the ad hoc committee's report, NIEHS established a standing ICCVAM "to implement a process by which new test methods of agency interest could be evaluated, and to coordinate interactions among agencies related to the development, validation, acceptance, and national and international harmonization of toxicological test methods."[5] In 2000, the ICCVAM Authorization Act established ICCVAM as a permanent interagency committee of NIEHS [6] and charged it:

> To establish, wherever feasible, guidelines, recommendations, and regulations that promote the regulatory acceptance of new or revised scientifically valid toxicological tests that protect human and animal health and the environment while reducing, refining, or replacing animal tests and ensuring human safety and product effectiveness (Public Law 106-545, 42 U.S.C. 285l-3).

Although reducing, refining, and replacing the use of animals in testing is an explicit focus of the ICCVAM mandate, scientific validation of new techniques hinges on demonstrating that the new methods are *relevant* and *reliable:* "Remember, the goal here is standardized testing methods that the agencies can require and that they can have confidence in the results of" (Interview S34). [7]

These requirements have shaped the efforts of NIEHS scientists to develop toxicogenomics. The next sections describe two specific efforts that aim to establish the relevance and reliability of microarray techniques. The first, phenotypic anchoring, addresses *relevance* by assessing "the ability of a test method to accurately measure or predict the endpoint, the biological activity of interest" (Interview S34). The second, the Toxicogenomics Research Consortium (TRC) is a research network that aims to address the issue of *reliability*, that is, the "reproducibility of that method within the laboratory and among other laboratories" (Interview S34). In both initiatives, the science of toxicogenomics is emerging in response to the requirements of the federal agencies charged with environmental governance.

"Let's Ground the New Technologies in the Old": Phenotypic Anchoring

The goal of phenotypic anchoring is to correlate gene expression profiles, produced in microarray analysis, with standard indices of toxicity, for example, from clinical chemistry or tissue pathology. In this way, phenotypic anchoring serves as a means of translation between toxicogenomics and standard toxicological tests; it makes linkages between molecular data and other levels of analysis. Administrators at the NIEHS articulate phenotypic anchoring as a way of grounding gene expression profiles in toxicological knowledge: "Let's ground the new technologies in the old, so that we know that as we replace them, they mean the same and our interpretations are correct" (Interview S39). Phenotypic anchoring thus directly addresses one requirement of regulatory adoption of alternative methods, namely, "a description of the relationship of new test measures to the range of responses in the standard test" [8] (ICCVAM 1997: 46).

Phenotypic anchoring is described by NIEHS scientists as a means to several interrelated ends. First, phenotypic anchoring is a means of ascertaining whether gene expression profiles can generate chemical-specific signatures, distinctive patterns that indicate known toxicological pathways and effects (Schmidt 2002). The goal of phenotypic anchoring is to establish correlations, that is, to be able to say that a given gene expression profile will correspond to a known index of toxicity: "We want to know that what the pathologist is telling you and what the gene expression profile is telling you [are] the same thing" (Field Notes, NIEHS July 2002). This aspect of phenotypic anchoring aims to establish equivalences between the knowledge products of genomics and those of traditional toxicology and pathology.

Second, researchers at the NCT regard phenotypic anchoring as a means of determining whether a change in a gene expression profile is toxicologically significant. Phenotypic anchoring is pursued as an objective and empirically grounded means of distinguishing evidence of toxicity from stochastic changes in gene expression profiles: "We are trying to make this as least subjective as possible, using histopathology, clinical chemistry, organ weight, and metabolites as the phenotypic anchorage of gene expression" (Field Notes, NIEHS July 2002). In the absence of data that establish the relationship between a gene expression pattern and a known physical or biochemical state, gene expression data are of unknown worth to risk assessment or regulation. Insofar as traditional toxicological measures provide the objective data to which toxicogenomics are compared, this aspect of phenotypic anchoring also serves as a means of translation between genomics, toxicology, and pathology.

Finally, phenotypic anchoring is a means of identifying genes whose expression may be induced by a given toxicant or class of toxicants. In this way, phenotypic anchoring is a kind of "discovery science"—a means of generating hypotheses for further scientific research. This is accomplished through establishing linkages between traditional indices of toxicology and gene expression profiles that, as such, translate between them. Thus, in each of these instances, phenotypic anchoring works as a means of translation between two toxicological languages. It links the quantitative data and gene expression profiles of toxicogenomics to the phenomenological data, clinical chemistry, and tissue specimens of traditional toxicology.

Successful phenotypic anchoring incorporates—that is, makes corporeal[9]—gene expression profile data. Phenotypic anchoring creates a chain of linkages among gene expression profiles, animal bodies, and human corporeality. This requires several steps. First, in correlating microarray data with tissue samples, organ sections, and so on, phenotypic anchoring established connections between the colorful spotted array of a gene expression profile and the actual bodies of animals used in traditional toxicological testing and risk assessment. Second, because animal bodies stand in for those of humans, phenotypic anchoring is a first step in establishing the relevance of toxicogenomic data for the health of human beings.

Through phenotypic anchoring, highly abstract genomic data are connected to human matters; they are linked to human bodies and populations. Thus, phenotypic anchoring is a means by which gene expression profiles and toxicogenomics are articulated with the "old-fashioned blood and guts toxicology" historically used by regulatory agencies (Interview P02).

Phenotypic anchoring as a mode of translation relies on the institutional connections between the NIEHS and the NTP, especially on the NTP's extensive archive of toxicological data. As this NTP scientist explained:

> There is a thirty year history of toxicology testing at NIEHS and the NTP. We've tested six hundred chemicals as thoroughly as they can be tested—two week, ninety day, and two year studies. Everything [is] done up to the state of the art. We've standardized feeding cycles, light cycles, dosing. We've done necropsy of forty tissues in mice and rats, males and females. . . . For each chemical, this takes seven to eight years, to go from testing to a blue book[10] (Interview S27).

The slides created during these 30 years of toxicology testing, the results of the necropsies on hundreds of thousands of animal bodies, and the reports of their clinical chemistry and histopathology are stored in an archive near the NIEHS campus. This archive contains the information on traditional toxicological indices needed for phenotypic anchoring and the incorporation of toxicogenomics.

Moreover, the NTP archive is invaluable for phenotypic anchoring because it contains the data from what many toxicologists regard as the gold standard of toxicology testing:

> The NTP is extremely rigorous—and it has to be. The NTP has to fulfill every aspect of good laboratory practice, because industry sends people over here to look through the lab books and try to find flaws. So, if there's a chance that the groups got messed up or some animals got the wrong dose, they'll contest the results. So, everything is carefully tracked and detailed. . . . The NTP does toxicology the right way (Interview S42).

In addition, the NTP has established many of the current standards of practice in contemporary toxicology testing.[11] The standardization of laboratory techniques used to assess the risks of carcinogens and the diagnostic terminology used in the interpretation of observed pathologies are regarded by many toxicologists as one of the most significant accomplishments of the NTP:

> The National Toxicology Program . . . is a real success story. If you think about that kind of testing, there are so many variables. They developed protocols for doing dosing, how to interpret results, and they've succeeded in having those interpretations adopted by both government and industry (Interview S27).

The NTP blue books are not only regarded as scientifically valid, they are also politically robust, as this toxicologist emphasized: "The NTP blue books are a bible. They are used by the regulatory agencies. They're the gold standard" (Interview S38).

Thus, while the NCT is using the NTP archive in the most material sense, that is, as a repository of the traditional indices of toxicity required to incorporate gene expression profiles, it also endeavors to use the archive in a much more expansive sense. Drawing on Foucault (1972), Gottweis (1995) conceptualizes an archive as "the general system of forming and transforming statements existing at a given period within a particular society." The NTP archive and the blue books based on the data it contains constitute the currently accepted system of forming and transforming statements about toxicological risks. Therefore, the credibility of gene expression profiles and, by extension, toxicogenomics rely on the success of phenotypic anchoring.

The NCT has also built a new, molecularized archive for toxicology and risk assessment, the Chemical Effects in Biological Systems (CEBS) database. This is a relational database that contains data from gene expression profiles, the NTP archives, the results of the phenotypic anchoring studies, and the standardization experiments of the TRC. The CEBS database, a project of the NCT, was shaped by three specific goals:

> (1) Create a reference toxicogenomic information system of studies on environmental chemicals/stressors and their effects; (2) Develop relational and descriptive compendia on toxicologically important genes, groups of genes, single nucleotide polymorphisms, mutants, and their functional phenotypes that are relevant to human health and environmental disease; (3) Create a toxicogenomics knowledge base to support hypothesis-driven research (NCT 2002: 25)

The CEBS database represents an attempt to create a new archive, a means of forming and transforming molecularized statements about toxicology, human health, and environmental disease. It endeavors to do this by bringing together new forms of knowledge (that is, knowledge about genes, groups of genes, single nucleotide polymorphisms, and mutations produced in toxicogenomics research) with *functional phenotypes*. These functional phenotypes are the artifacts that populate the NTP archive and thus provide linkages between gene expression profiles and traditional indices of toxicity.

As with phenotypic anchoring techniques, the CEBS database is a means of translating between toxicogenomics and traditional toxicology, between molecular grammars based *in silico* microarrays and those that rely on animal bioassays. This is undertaken, in part, by creating an interface between the CEBS database and the NTP archives. The goal is to enable researchers to link the gene expression profiles data in the CEBS with "all the National Toxicology Program has done on the acute toxicity of over 500 chemicals" (Interview S39). Such linkages would allow researchers to call up both sets of data with one relational query of the database. Put differently, CEBS will answer a user's question in two languages and provide a means of translating between them. Indeed, the CEBS provides "dictionaries and explanatory text" to "guide researchers in understanding toxicogenomics databases" (NCT 2002: 26). The CEBS database also links to other genomics and proteomic resources on the Web, "providing users the suite of information and tools needed to fully interpret toxicogenomics data" (NCT 2002: 26). Thus, the CEBS is a translational resource for environmental health scientists who want to make statements about environmental health and illness using molecular techniques.

Standardizing the Grammar: The Toxicogenomics Research Consortium

At the same time, the TRC, an extramural research initiative of the NCT, endeavors to standardize this new, molecular toxicological grammar.[12] The TRC was established in November 2001, when the NIEHS awarded grants to five institutions to participate as cooperative research members (CRM) of the NCT. The initial goal of the TRC is "to conduct a series of cooperative gene expression experiments using shared and complementary microarray platforms" (NCT 2002: 14). The purpose of the cooperative experiments is to "develop standard operating procedures and quality control standards for gene expression experiments and to develop technology standards and bioinformatics tools for data comparison across the CRM" (NCT 2002: 14). The development of these standards and bioinformatics tools, in turn, will allow the gene expression profiles generated by TRC members to be submitted to the CEBS database, where it will contribute to the initial collection of toxicogenomic data available for public query.

The TRC project thus endeavors to maximize the usability of the CEBS in particular and of toxicogenomics in general as resources for making molecularized toxicological statements. As this toxicologist made clear, a new archive requires user guides and ways of "learning the rules" of its organization:

> What does the data mean? That's the big question. There is so much data. It's like being given the Encyclopedia Britannica and ten seconds to find an answer. . . . You know the answer is in there somewhere, but you have to learn the rules or what volume to go to, and you have to learn the rule within that volume. Where do you look it up? And you have to learn the rules for not only reading what's there, but understanding and interpreting. . . . (Interview S35).

For toxicogenomics to be able to travel widely, such user guides must be standardized and widely accepted as reliable (Bowker & Star 2000; Timmermans & Berg 1997). The TRC works to accomplish this standardization and to create a consistent, usable molecular grammar for toxicology.

The TRC also enrolls scientists (and presumably their postdoctoral fellow and graduate students) at five major environmental health research centers, creating a network of active participants in the establishment of toxicogenomics as a standardized, usable molecular toxicological science. This is especially important insofar as "the external scientific community's participation is essential to the certification of new knowledge and its incorporation into policy" (Jasanoff 1990: 206).

Regulating Molecular Events

As noted in the 1997 ICCVAM report, regulatory agencies tend to be conservative in their orientation to alternative toxicological methods and "do not readily accept new and revised test methods" (ICCVAM 1997: 45). In interviews, environmental health scientists made similar observations, commenting, for example, that "once the regulatory community develops some tools that give it confidence about the nature of its decisions, I think they tend to hold on tenaciously to those tools" (Interview S95). A toxicologist stated bluntly that "the people who do this, they don't want to do new methods. They have already bought the equipment to do the old methods" (Interview S13). As an EPA scientist observed, "there is certainly a lag time between the appearance of the data and its ability to be used in regulatory decision making" (Interview P14).

EPA officials state clearly, "Agency scientists don't have blinders on and they know this [genomics] is happening . . . it doesn't take a rocket toxicologist to figure out that this is going to be a big deal," but they acknowledge that there is much work to be done to ensure that the Agency will be "ready when the future comes" (Interview P03).[13] To date, the EPA has issued two formal statements about its position regarding the uses of genomics in environmental risk assessment and regulation.[14] Both emphasize the need for precisely the kind of research initiated by NIEHS scientists working on phenotypic anchoring and with the TRC. Phenotypic anchoring is critical because "most substances currently are regulated on frank toxicity rather than on a molecular level response" (EPA 2004: 19). Therefore, integrating genomic information into regulatory review at EPA requires that "the link between molecular indicator, exposure, and adverse outcome . . . be established" (EPA 2004: 30). In fact, the EPA has identified "linking genomics information to adverse outcomes" as a primary research challenge "that must be addressed before genomics data can provide information essential to the support of risk assessment and regulatory decision making" (EPA 2004: 40). Likewise, among the research needs identified by the EPA is to "establish reproducibility and consistency of data" from molecular profiling techniques (EPA 2004: 30). According to the EPA, standardization of "experimental design and data analysis for genomics" and the "development of data quality standards based on performance of microarrays" is necessary to "enhance the reproducibility of results and the reliability of conclusions drawn from these data" (EPA 2004: 4). These are precisely the foci of the TRC.

NIEHS scientists, informed by the Institute's participation in the ICC-VAM process and their previous experience providing data to regulatory agencies, skillfully anticipated what research would be crucial to regulatory acceptance of microarray techniques. Consequently, years before the EPA formally articulated its specific research needs vis-à-vis genomics, NIEHS scientists and their allies implemented research agendas that address them. In this way, the requirements of the regulatory process—and the social and political concerns embedded within them—have been an inextricable part of the development of the science of toxicogenomics.

As noted in previous chapters, environmental health scientists understand their research to be in the service of protecting public health, principally by providing an empirical basis for public policy. Initiatives such as phenotypic anchoring and the TRC clearly demonstrate that environmental health research may be strongly oriented to meeting legislative and procedural requirements. However, environmental health scientists also have begun efforts to transform the regulatory process itself. While toxicogenomics provided an early focus for such efforts, they now encompass multi-institute initiatives to molecularize environmental regulation.

MAKING A MOLECULAR REGULATORY SCIENCE

In 2004, the EPA's white paper on genomics called for "a multi-stakeholder process to ensure scientific consensus around the understanding of adverse effects based on genomics data" (EPA 2004: 15). The NIEHS has taken a leadership role in engaging stakeholders, including "the chemical and pharmaceutical manufacturing industries, the green groups, environmental groups, and consumer groups, the Environmental Defense Fund, the EPA, FDA, and other regulatory agencies, and policymakers... staffers from Congress" (Interview S39).

Efforts to build a broad consensus among stakeholders about the meanings and applications of genomics are predicated on the assumption that new and better scientific techniques will provide a means for transcending the scientific uncertainties, political conflicts, and litigation that often characterize environmental health risk assessment and regulation in the United States. Some environmental health scientists challenge this assumption, suggesting, "As long as we define the issue of risk assessment and the risk management process as a legalistic process under an adversarial legal system, I don't see any major improvements." (Interview S13). In fact, there is no evidence that advances in scientific knowledge "predictably correlate with reductions or increases in policy conflict" in the environmental health arena (Jasanoff 1990); rather, insofar as the formal adversarial style of American regulatory decision making remains unchanged by the incorporation of molecular data, one would expect ongoing controversy and contestation. However, scientists' framing of the limitations of current risk assessment techniques—the consensus critique—provides a shared point of departure for many of the stakeholders participating in the consensus-building process.

Moreover, irrespective of whether they produce a politically robust consensus about the uses of genomic data in risk assessment, consensus-building efforts already have had two important consequences vis-à-vis the diffusion of genomic techniques. First, these efforts have provided a forum for social learning about genomic technologies, with regulators from different federal agencies learning from each other, as well as from laboratory scientists, about genomic technologies. Second, they have provided a rationale for collaborative research and development efforts that now officially link the research agendas of the National Institutes of Health (and especially the NIEHS) and the EPA in an effort to transform environmental health protection.

Building Consensus . . .

From the perspective of the NIEHS leadership, the goals of consensus building are to "to define the environment" in which toxicogenomics is introduced to the stakeholders and to establish agreement regarding the meaning and appropriate uses of genomic data in advance of any specific regulatory review:

> I just want the technologies to have as full an impact in as short of
> a period as possible. And without the kind of things that we are do-
> ing to educate stakeholders, policy makers, and the American public,

regulatory agencies will not be allowed to use [the new technologies], even when they decide to use them. So we have just got to bring along everybody to make sure that if three years down the road we can predict toxicity, by gosh let's do it then and let's not wait x number of years for everybody else to catch up (Interview S37).

Toward these ends, in 2001, the NIEHS asked the National Academy of Sciences (NAS) to establish a Committee on Emerging Issues and Data on Environmental Contaminants.

The NAS is well positioned to facilitate this process because of its reputation for scientific excellence, neutrality, and objectivity in bringing closure to scientific debates.[15] As one NIEHS scientist put it:

> The National Academy of Science is supposed to be the pure, above reproach group. They have no stake in this. They are just trying to be the honest broker. So they are going to bring people around the table and they're going to let them argue and debate and finally get a consensus (Interview S27).

The significant scientific prestige and credibility of the NAS are also of value in the translation of toxicogenomics. As this environmental health scientist noted, "any significant NAS report or workshop . . . can signal the official definition of a field" (Field Notes, NIEHS July 2002). This may be particularly true in regard to risk assessment, because the National Research Council (NRC) of the NAS wrote *Risk Assessment in the Federal Government: Managing the Process*. Referred to by insiders as "the Red Book" (Interview P05; Keller 2009: 146), this serves as "the Bible" at the federal agencies (Interview P05) where it provides "a common starting point for everybody in risk assessment" (Interview P03).[16]

Unlike many NAS committees, which are charged with undertaking studies and producing a consensus report to answer a specific scientific question, the initial committee sponsored by the NIEHS—the Committee on Emerging Issues and Data on Environmental Contaminants (hereafter the Committee)—was designed to serve as "a forum for discussion":

> The goals are to bring issues to the forefront, to identify issues, and . . . holding symposia to focus on those particular issues, so that more issues can be identified or discussed, and different viewpoints can be brought

up. Then also, to develop ideas where more specific attention might be needed, either by future NAS studies or other mechanisms (Interview S59).

The original Committee membership included environmental health scientists, lawyers, a scientist from the National Resources Defense Council, and representatives from the Chemical Industry Institute for Toxicology and various chemical, pharmaceutical, and biotechnology companies.[17] According to the NIEHS leadership, the goal of the Committee was to

> ... bring together all the stakeholders in the field: industry, scientists, lay public, unions, policy makers, environmental groups, regulatory agencies. We want to get everyone around the table to talk about toxicogenomic data, to develop case studies to explore how the data can be used (Interview S39).

These case studies, then, were to provide a means of producing "blueprints" for the use of toxicogenomics by the regulatory agencies. As a toxicologist explained:

> There will be all of these position papers with all these case studies, and the cases will become reality with time. So the EPA and the FDA won't have to say, "Toxicogenomics, what is that? What does this mean? And how do I use it?" They've already got a blueprint that they've agreed to and everybody's agreed to and they've been informed (Interview S37).

In addition to providing guidance to the regulatory agencies, the NAS committee process was designed to allow traditionally adversarial groups—and especially the industries regulated by the federal agencies—to "participate with government" in the process of making decisions about toxicogenomics so that they know that "government acted responsibly" in developing the technology and its applications in risk assessment and regulation:

> The concern is that every time there is a peak [in expression] in the data, the environmental groups will react. Or that every time there is a question about how to interpret, that industry will say the data means nothing. So, we need to get this group of people together to set

standards up front. So, when we get data, we've agreed about how it will be used and it can be used immediately, so that we won't have to wait 5–10 years (Interview S58).

This approach is congruent with the focus of the consensus critique on the process—rather than the outcomes—of risk assessment.

From 2001 to 2007, the Committee held a series of workshops focused on issues central to the translation and validation of toxicogenomics.[18] When the Committee completed its charge, the NAS established a new standing Committee on the Use of Emerging Science for Environmental Health Decisions to provide "a public venue for communication among government, industry, environmental groups, and the academic community about scientific advances in methods and approaches that can be used in the identification, quantification and control of environmental impacts on human health" and to "consider issues on the use of emerging science for environmental health decisions."[19] Although the mandate of the new committee extends beyond toxicogenomics, it is meant to "build on recent NRC reports on toxicity testing and toxicogenomics and . . . explore new developments in toxicology, molecular biology, bioinformatics, and related fields."[20]

Concomitantly, two other NAS committees also were envisioning the future of toxicological testing and risk assessment. At the suggestion of the Committee on Emerging Issues and Data on Environmental Contaminants, the NRC supported a committee charged specifically with considering "applications of toxicogenomic technologies to predictive toxicology." This committee authored a report entitled *Applications of Toxicogenomic Technologies to Predictive Toxicology and Risk Assessment* (NRC 2007a). Beginning in 2004, the EPA sponsored a Committee on Toxicity Testing and Assessment of Environmental Agents, which authored a report entitled *Toxicity Testing in the 21st Century: A Vision and a Strategy* (NRC 2007b). Echoing the earlier committee's focus on how toxicogenomics can improve risk assessment and regulation, the reports of these committees highlight the potential of "advances in molecular biology, biotechnology and other fields" to "illuminate changes at the molecular level" in "samples . . . of human origin," thereby making toxicity testing "quicker, less expensive, and more directly relevant to human exposures" (NRC 2007b).

. . . from Critique

Consensus-building efforts have been facilitated by the fact that even stakeholders who vehemently and litigiously disagree about the outcomes of specific risk assessments and regulatory decisions concur with the consensus critique regarding the process by which chemicals currently are tested and regulated. Chapter 2 described how environmental health scientists have diagnosed the limitations of the risk assessment process, focusing particularly on the expense, time, and uncertainties inherent to the two-year rodent cancer bioassay. Scientists argue that these limitations lead to bottlenecks in testing and to an extensive backlog of chemicals waiting to be assessed. ICCVAM formalizes a component of this critique with its mandate to reduce, replace, or refine the use of animals in toxicological testing (ICCVAM 1997: 20). Lastly, multiple stakeholders frame "unproductive legal and scientific battles" as a problematic and unproductive dynamic that is too often a part of environmental health regulation (Balbus 2008:47). Together, these critiques constitute a "policy narrative" (Stone 1989; Keller 2009) positing that molecular techniques will remediate long-standing challenges in environmental health regulation and policy making. As noted by sociologists, careful framings can facilitate the translation of practices from one site to another (Strang & Soule 1998: 277). Here, the consensus critique provides disparate and often antagonistic stakeholders with some shared criteria for deliberating the appropriate uses of genomics in environmental risk assessment and regulation. It also aligns new molecular practices and data with existing normative assumptions about the need for more biologically based and precise means of doing environmental health risk assessment and regulation, thereby imbuing novel molecular techniques with extant cultural understandings of appropriate and effective regulatory action.

The regulatory agencies have been remarkably receptive to this narrative. The EPA's official statements on genomics for risk assessment and regulatory applications invoke the consensus critique. Nearly one-third of the EPA's *Interim Policy on Genomics* is devoted to affirming the Agency's belief that genomics "will ultimately improve the quality of information used in the risk assessment process" by identifying "variability and susceptibility," providing "a better understanding of the mechanism or mode of action," reducing or eliminating "traditional types of toxicity testing," evaluating "cumulative impact," and "ultimately reduce the uncertainties in the assessment of hazard, exposure, and risk from stressors" (EPA 2002: 3). In its white paper on genomics, the EPA avers that, although genomics will not "fundamentally alter the risk assessment process," it is "expected to serve as a more powerful tool for evaluating the exposure and effects of environmental stressors" (2004: 4).[21] Here again, the EPA highlights mode of action, susceptible populations, and chemical mixtures as key issues in risk assessment that genomic information might productively address (2004: 17–29).

Additionally, by bringing together diverse stakeholders around a shared agenda (and effacing their substantive political differences), the consensus-building process has had two structural effects. First, consensus committees provide a sort of "organized pedagogy" (Simmons, Dobbin, & Garrett 2008: 31), in which stakeholders learn not only about new practices and the data they produce, but also about how relevant actors are adopting these practices. As noted in previous sociological research, the intensity of contact among officials is associated with policy diffusion, as actors can learn not only directly from their own experiences, but also from the policy experiments of others (Simmons, Dobbin, & Garrett 2008: 25). EPA scientists emphasize particularly that they are watching and learning from their colleagues at the FDA, where pharmacogenomic data have more quickly become a part of the regulatory review of pharmaceuticals: "[E]verybody is looking to pharmaceuticals as the place where the technology will immediately find a home . . . " (Interview P02; see also Balbus 2008; FDA 2005).[22]

At the same time, building on the consensus critique, the reports issued by the NAS/NRC committees have called for coordinated funding efforts, public-private partnerships, and collaborations among government, academia, and the private sector in order to realize these goals. Indeed, among the recommendations of the report specifically focused on toxicogenomics was "a coordinated effort approaching the scale of the human genome project" (NRC 2007a: 4).

In 2008, the Department of Health and Human Services (DHHS) and the EPA issued a Memorandum of Understanding (MOU) for a collaboration among the NTP, EPA, and the National Institutes of Health Chemical Genomics Center (NCGC) aimed at advancing the "evolution of toxicology" by developing "methods for toxicology testing that are more scientifically and economically efficient and models for risk assessment that are more biologically based" (EPA 2008: 1). The article in *Science* that announced the collaboration opened with a recounting of the "theoretical rationale" provided by the work of the NRC (Collins, Gray, & Bucher 2008: 906). By developing high-throughput screening assays (e.g., *in vitro* techniques such as microarrays), investigating variations in susceptibility to exposures, and developing new methods for computational toxicology, this new transagency collaboration is expected to "generate data more relevant to humans; expand the number of chemicals that are tested; and reduce the time, money, and number of animals involved in testing" (NIH 2008). The overarching goal of the collaboration is no less than "transforming environmental health protection" using *molecular* techniques (Collins, Gray, & Bucher 2008: 906).

As noted in articles describing this proposed transformation of environmental health risk assessment and regulation, the concept of adding more mechanistic data to risk assessment is not new (Schmidt 2009: 350). However, the proposals published by the NRC in 2007, and the MOU and implementation plans developed by the NIH and EPA following, go beyond adding new data into the old system of assessing the risks of environmental chemicals. Rather, these efforts, which scientists have dubbed *Tox21*, endeavor to transform toxicology "from a system based on whole animal testing to one founded primarily on *in vitro* methods that evaluate changes in biologic processes using cells, cell lines, or cellular components, preferably of human origin" (NRC 2007b:1). The goal here is thoroughly molecularized system of environmental risk assessment and regulation.

THE FUTURE PERFECT?

This chapter has described the diffusion of high-throughput sequencing techniques to the environmental health sciences and examined scientists' efforts to promote their uptake in environmental health risk assessment and regulation. Focusing particularly on the diffusion of toxicogenomics, I have described the importance of structural connections, such as the relationships between NHGRI and NIEHS scientists, and of culturally mediated processes of connecting, such as the efforts of NIEHS scientists to translate, standardize, and build consensus regarding the meaning of toxicogenomics data.

At the same time, the chapter has explored how efforts to build consensus around the applications of genomic data in risk assessment and regulation have shaped the emergence and diffusion of genomic research in the environmental health sciences. Specifically, the science of toxicogenomics has emerged in and through research initiatives aimed at facilitating its uptake by the regulatory agencies, especially the EPA. Both research on phenotypic anchoring and the standardization efforts of the TRC reflect and are responsive to the ICCVAM process that governs the validation of alternative toxicological testing methods. Consequently, the requirements of environmental risk assessment and regulation have shaped the development of toxicogenomics. Likewise, the contentious and litigious politics of the environmental health arena have entered into the emergence of toxicogenomics, especially in NIEHS-funded efforts to build consensus about the meaning of gene expression profiles, other forms of molecular data, and their appropriate uses in environmental risk assessment and regulation.

Scientists and regulators are deploying similar strategies in Tox21. Alongside detailed plans for scientific research to identify the relevant molecular "toxicity pathways," Tox21 implementation plans call for efforts to build stakeholders' trust in new technologies (Firestone et al. 2010: 156). Toward this end, the EPA is promoting a model of validation and consensus building nearly identical to that used for toxicogenomics. First, it emphasizes the importance of "grounding the science" in relation to the current standard techniques. Second, it envisions a series of "periodic workshops," in which stakeholders come together to work through a series of case studies well in advance of the deployment of the technologies in regulatory decision making (Firestone et al. 2010). Against narratives emphasizing that environmental health science is conducted to meet the needs of the regulatory agencies, we see here how *environmental health scientists endeavor to transform the agencies' understanding of the science they need.*

Critical to such efforts is the consensus critique, with its array of complaints about current risk assessment practices. Often policy narratives focus on specific social problems; here, the focus is on the policy-making process itself. To be sure, stakeholders continue to disagree about whether "overinterpretation" leading to excessive regulation or the weakening of regulations is the primary danger posed by incorporating genomics into risk assessment (Balbus 2008: 47; Phillips 2008: 36). Nonetheless, the consensus critique provides a major rationale for the molecularization of environmental health risk assessment and regulation. By bringing together stakeholders and providing them with a shared focus, the consensus critique has facilitated social learning about new technologies among the regulatory agencies and fostered the development of new collaborative networks and initiatives devoted to a molecular revolution in toxicological testing.

The centrality of the consensus critique to this process is also important, as we will see, to understanding the critical response of environmental justice activists to molecular genetic and genomic technologies. The consensus critique represents an effort to scientize the challenges of environmental health governance, asserting that "there are systematic, discoverable methods" for addressing controversy and conflict about environmental regulation and suggesting that these methods can be developed and applied independently of stakeholders' social and political interests (Jasanoff 1996: 173). In the following chapter, I demonstrate how environmental justice activists' critical responses to genomics may help us see the social, economic, and political concerns that remain unaddressed in efforts to use molecular techniques to improve risk assessment and regulation and advance population health.

SIX The Molecular Is Political

To the question "is it genes or is it the environment?"
I would say that the answer is "Neither, it's politics and
power."

Environmental Justice Activist, WEACT Conference,
February 2002

In 2002, five mothers, on behalf of their fourteen children, brought suit
against the owner of an 86-year-old apartment complex in Greenwood,
Mississippi, where they lived, and National Lead Industries, Inc., one
of the largest paint manufacturers in the United States. The plaintiffs
in the case, *Tamiko Jones, et al., v. NL Industries, et al.* (Civil Action No.
4:03CV229), claimed that their children had been poisoned by the lead
in the paint on the walls and, as a consequence, had suffered irreversible
mental damage, including loss of IQ, impaired cognitive function, and
behavioral problems. The defendants argued that the children's genetic

An earlier version of this analysis appeared as Shostak, S. "Environmental Justice and
Genomics: Acting on the Futures of Environmental Health." *Science as Culture* 13(4): 539-562.
Copyright (2004) Taylor & Francis.

inheritances were the primary cause of their conditions, rather than exposure to lead.

All fourteen of the children involved in the case had documented blood lead levels above 10 μg/dL, a level of lead exposure that multiple scientific studies have found to be associated with impairments in cognitive function, fetal organ development, intelligence, hearing, and behavior difficulties. Three of the children had lead measurements over three times that amount. According to their doctor's records, several of the children had elevated lead levels for many years. *All* of the environmental health scientists who testified or submitted affidavits to the court supported the claims being made by the mothers of the children about the effects of lead on their behavior and cognitive functioning.

Given that low-income and minority children are more likely to be exposed to lead and to suffer from lead poisoning (Lanphear et al. 1998), children growing up in Greenwood, Mississippi, are unquestionably a high-risk population. Greenwood is located in Leflore County, where the percentage of people living below the poverty line is 42.4%, more than twice the average for the rest of the state (20.7%), and three times the national average (13.0%).[1] The median household income in Leflore County is only $24,568, lagging well behind the state and national averages (respectively, $36,424 and $50,740). Nearly 71% of the county's population is African American (compared to 37.2% in the state and 12.8% nationally).[2] Sherry Wragg, the mother of four of the young plaintiffs in the suit, was very clear about the role of poverty and lack of opportunity in her family's situation. She told a reporter from the Associated Press that she had looked for alternative housing but could not afford to move herself and her four children from their 1.5-bedroom residence on "the little income I have" (Byrd 2006a).

The defendants in the case offered another set of explanations for the cognitive and behavioral problems of the children noted in the suit. They argued that the cause of the children's impairments was not lead exposure, but rather their families' histories of mental retardation, learning disabilities, and behavioral problems. Among the expert witnesses retained by the defendants was Barbara Quinton, a geneticist and former director of the Medical Genetics Clinic at Howard University, who reviewed the children's medical records and performed medical exams (Quinton 2005a). Quinton then recommended that several of the children undergo genetic and chromosomal testing for conditions, including fragile X syndrome, associated with impaired cognitive function and behavioral problems.

All of the genetic and chromosomal analyses ordered by Quinton were negative. During the trial she testified that *none of the children had an identifiable genetic syndrome* (Quinton 2005b: 29). Nonetheless, Quinton claimed that the family pedigree "itself is a test that is very important in this regard" (Quinton 2005b: 33). Based on her assessment of the family pedigrees she had assembled, Quinton testified that the children's cognitive deficits and other problems were "polygenetic," that is, caused by "a collection of multiple genes" producing "familial mild mental retardation" (Quinton 2005b: 33). In fact, Quinton suggested that mild familial mental retardation had so compromised the children's IQ that, even if they did suffer the 1–3 point reductions in IQ associated with blood lead levels of 10 (μg/dL), this damage would not have a functional effect on their abilities.

Witnesses for the defendants were clearly aware that the children were growing up poor and disadvantaged. Colleen Parker, a professor of pediatrics at the University of Mississippi Medical Center, testified that "economic deprivation" contributed to the children's impairments. However, rather than acknowledging the extensive evidence that low-income children are at increased risk for lead poisoning, Parker argued that factors such as "familial history of retardation, poor environmental stimulation, and economic deprivation" explained the children's cognitive and behavioral impairments[3] (Case 4:03-cv-00229-MPM, Document 246: 6). As noted by the Court, *none* of the experts retained by the defendants had expertise regarding lead poisoning in children.

After a three-week trial, the jury in *Tamiko Jones, et al., v. NL Industries, et al.* returned a verdict in favor of the apartment owner and the lead industry. The attorney representing the mothers and their children attributed the verdict to the success of the defendants in convincing the jury that the paint used in their apartments might not be the primary cause of the children's ailments: "We talked to the jury and they couldn't conclude that the paint was the major cause of these kids' conditions" (Byrd 2006b). Thus, the children were found to be victims of unidentified genetic factors, rather than measured environmental exposures known to be associated with their symptoms.

The *Tamiko Jones, et al.* case is not an anomaly. In recent years, blaming children's genetic inheritance has become a popular strategy of lead companies in toxic tort cases (Byrd 2006a; see also Markowitz & Rosner 2002; Oreskes & Conway 2010). More broadly, defendants in a variety of toxic tort cases have argued that the health problems of African American plaintiffs are caused by "hereditary health problems among blacks" rather than chemical exposures (Capek 1993). To date, defendants' genetic claims are rarely substantiated with data from genetic tests; rather, as in the *Tamiko Jones, et al.* case, defendants rely on hired medical experts who make general claims about the relationships between heredity and health outcomes in order to discredit plaintiffs' arguments about the health effects of environmental exposures (Hoffman & Rothenberg 2007).[4]

Although gene-environment interaction has not been directly implicated in these cases, such uses of genetic arguments by defendants in toxic tort cases—and especially their broad claims about purported "hereditary health problems" among African-Americans—are critical to understanding the response of environmental justice (EJ) activists to the ascendance of molecular genetic research in the environmental health sciences. Simply put, these arguments highlight how genetics can be used to undermine claims about the role of environmental exposures in causing mental and physical impairments. At the same time, they point to the potential of genetics to reify race as a biological category, while directing attention away from the social, economic, and political dimensions of race that contribute, for example, to the higher rates of lead poisoning among poor children of color. Both of these possibilities are of great concern to EJ activists and the communities of color on whose behalf they advocate.

This chapter examines the perspectives of EJ activists. These perspectives are important both because EJ activists are active stakeholders in the environmental health arena and because they offer a contrasting analysis of its central concerns. Environmental health scientists and regulators identify EJ activists as among the "key stakeholders" with whom they must "build bridges" in establishing a role for molecular genetic and genomic technologies in environmental risk assessment and policy making

(Interview S39). However, building such bridges poses myriad challenges. Most fundamentally, scientists and activists have very different understandings of the causes of environmentally associated disease and therefore very different visions of the most effective strategies for preventing illness. Relatedly, scientists and activists differ in their definitions of the key challenges in the environmental health arena. However, EJ activists also articulate a number of specific concerns about genetic research in the environmental health sciences, including the possibilities that it will reinforce biological conceptualizations of race, divert critical resources from efforts to identify and ameliorate exposures, and obfuscate the social, political, and economic factors that make poor communities of color more likely to be exposed to chemical hazards. Simply put, EJ activists call attention to the possibility that genetics research will "blame the victims" and "let the polluters off the hook" (WEACT 2002: 66). The critiques of EJ activists thereby raise questions about the social and political implications of scientists' efforts to define, operationalize, and govern the environment at the molecular level; particularly, they ask us to consider the consequences of molecularization for our ability to understand and address the dimensions of social structure, such as racism and political power, that shape the distribution of environmental health and illness in the United States.

ENVIRONMENTAL HEALTH, JUSTICE,
AND THE LIMITS OF SCIENCE

The Environmental Justice Movement in the United States

In the late 1970s and early 1980s, a new kind of environmental activism began to emerge across the United States. Most often originating in working-class neighborhoods and communities of color burdened by toxic exposures, citizens began to challenge the inequitable distribution of environmental hazards and their effects (Bullard 1994: 8). This activism varied by community context: "In the white working-class community, it took the form of 'citizen-worker' or 'anti-toxics' movement . . . in communities of color, it took the form of the 'People of Color Environmental Movement'" (Pellow & Brulle 2005: 8). EJ activists drew on both the institutional and ideological resources of the American Civil Rights movement and a variety of contemporary movements focused on the environment and health (Bryant & Hockman 2005). Insofar as it has extended the focus of the environmental movement from conservation and protection of nature to concern about inequality in environmental exposures and their deleterious consequences, the EJ movement has challenged American society to redefine its conception of what constitutes the environment and how it is relevant to public health (Pellow & Brulle 2005: 8). The EJ movement especially has called attention to the unequal burden of environmental hazards borne by people of color.[5]

In 1991, at the First National People of Color Environmental Leadership Summit, EJ activists refined both the mission and the infrastructure of their growing movement. Activists at this meeting drafted Principles for Environmental Justice that called for resisting "the taking of our lands and communities" as well as "the strict enforcement of the principles of informed consent, and a halt to the testing of experimental . . . medical procedures . . . on people of color" (WEACT 2002). Participants at the Summit also articulated the need for greater institutional coordination among local groups. Subsequently, environmental justice activists have organized strategic geographically-based networks[6] and national constituency-based networks.[7] Participating organizations work together to share and develop agendas, strategies, and tactics oriented to "protect[ing] the environment and health of all, including those living in communities of color and places that are economically exploited" (Shepard et al. 2002).

The central foci of the EJ movement have changed during the course of its development. Initially, EJ activists focused on environmental racism, defined as "racial discrimination in environmental policymaking, the enforcement of regulations and laws, the deliberate targeting of communities of color for toxic waste facilities, the official sanctioning of the life-threatening presence of poisons and pollutants in our communities, and the history of excluding people of color from leadership of the ecology movements" (in Brulle & Pellow 2006: 105). However, activists soon broadened their framing to *environmental injustice,* defined as the disproportionate burden of environmental hazards on specific social groups.

The EJ movement has been successful in developing and promulgating environmental justice as a framework for identifying unfair, unjust, and inequitable conditions and decisions. In 1994, President Bill Clinton signed Executive Order 12898, which states that:

> To the greatest extent practicable and permitted by law . . . each Federal agency shall make achieving environmental justice part of its mission by identifying and addressing, as appropriate, disproportionately high and adverse human health and/or environmental effects of its programs, policies and activities on minority populations and low income populations in the United States . . . (Section 1-101).[8]

However, in 2004, the Inspector General of the EPA found that the agency was not doing an effective job of enforcing environmental justice: "[T]he EPA has no strategic plans, goals, or performance measures designed to advance the intent of this Executive Order . . . " (Pellow & Brulle 2005: 10). In recent years, both scholars and activists have observed that neither the many local victories of EJ groups nor the establishment of EJ offices at the federal agencies have resulted in significant progress in addressing the broader social processes relevant to ecological protection and social justice (Pellow & Brulle 2005).

EJ activists rely on individual and organizational donors, foundation support, and government funding for their work. From the perspective of foundation funding, the EJ movement may be "the most underfunded social movement in the United States"; from 1996 to 1999, it received less than 5% of all environmental funding given by foundations nationwide (Faber & McCarthy 2001: i).[9] Federal funding is also available to organizations working on environmental justice issues. The EPA's Office of Environmental Justice has competitive grants programs at the local, state, and regional levels. From 1994 to 2009, the EPA's Environmental Justice Small Grants Program awarded $20 million to 1,130 community-based, local, and tribal organizations working with communities disproportionately impacted by environmental harms and risks.[10] A second EPA initiative, the Collaborative Problem-Solving Cooperative Agreements Program, provides funding to community groups to use EPA's Environmental Justice Collaborative Problem-Solving Model in order to "provide communities with information to help them develop proactive, strategic, and visionary approaches to address environmental justice issues, and to achieve community health and sustainability."[11] Starting in the mid-1990s, the NIEHS provided extramural funding via two programs that promote community engagement in environmental health research and intervention, the Environmental Justice: Partnerships for Communication Program and the Community-Based Participatory Research (CBPR) Program.[12]

Practically, this means that EJ activists are stakeholders in the budgetary and grant-making processes of major federal scientific and regulatory agencies. Indeed, as seen in Chapter 1, Peggy Shepard, the founder and executive director of West Harlem Environmental Action (WEACT), an environmental justice group based in Northern Manhattan, was one of five individuals called on by the Congressional Committee on Oversight and Government Reform to testify about changes in the research priorities of the NIEHS. Members of EJ organizations have served on the community advisory boards for major environmental research projects and on grant review committees (Interview P01). Despite these forms of engagement, the environmental justice frame tends to highlight the limitations of scientific methods in addressing EJ issues.

Defining the Problem: Social Justice Versus Scientific Uncertainty

The EJ movement has a complex relationship to science, which some activists characterize as a "double edged sword" (Akaba 2004). This complexity derives from the dual—indeed, opposed—stances that the movement takes in relation to scientific research: "On the one hand, the movement represents a broad challenge to the authority of scientific knowledge . . . on the other hand, the outcomes of local struggles are often dependent on the regulatory regimes that structure environmental assessment and on the knowledge practices and disciplinary commitments that feed mainstream environmental health research" (Frickel 2011: 24).

Several significant dynamics push EJ activists away from engaging with science. To begin, the environmental justice perspective emphasizes

civil rights, fair and fully participatory democratic decision-making processes, and respect for grassroots knowledge (Capek 1993: 8); it thereby
defines environmental concerns as civil rights, social justice, and human
rights issues, rather than as scientific or technical matters. Second, although environmental justice activists may begin their efforts with faith
in the unbiased and apolitical nature of science and in the inherent fairness of the regulatory process, research suggests that participating in this
process tends to erode their confidence. For example, activists recount
watching "expensive scientists" and lawyers use "highly technical data"
to invalidate the "anecdotes" of citizens living in exposed communities
(Capek 1993: 15), leading to disappointment with science "because it
often . . . discounts their experiences" (Ellis 2004). Consequently, science
appears, to many, as "an arena in which our opponents have the upper
hand . . . science has been used by industry and the government, typically
against our interests and safety" (Akaba 2004). Further, activists have encountered scientific norms regarding standards of evidence, timelines,
peer review and publication as barriers to working even with scientists
who are supportive of their goals[13] (Allen 2004). Lastly, in expressing
concerns about science, EJ activists point to a history of outrages, including the abuse of research subjects from communities of color and the use
of (now widely disproven) racial science as rationales for discrimination
and abuse.[14] Therefore, activists say that they question whether "scientists have . . . their agenda all on the up and up, or their heart in the
right place?" (Field Notes, New York 2002). Some state emphatically that
they "don't believe that the mainstream research model has any place in
the environmental justice movement" (Larson 2004). More generally, as
a longtime EJ activist told me in one of my earliest interviews, "there is
a lot of skepticism about science" in the EJ Movement (Field Notes, San
Francisco 2001; see also Montague 2004).

At the same time, many EJ activists recognize that scientific research
has been a "key tool in the struggle for environmental and social justice"
insofar as it has "provided much of the evidence community activists
use to bolster claims of disproportionate environmental impacts on poor
communities of color" (Ellis 2004). Indeed, even though the movement's
claims are located squarely within a discourse of civil rights, the outcomes

of community-level struggles often depend on the generation of credible evidence regarding the dynamics of exposure to chemicals and their biological effects (Frickel 2011). Consequently, EJ activists argue that when science is "taken back"—that is, when it is put in the service of movement goals—"it can also be a powerful tool to equalize the playing field and bolster our struggles for safe and healthy environments" (Akaba 2004). Related, they contend that when scientific data are analyzed in collaboration with EJ activists, who bring especially a sensitivity to issues of race and class, research can be "made accountable" to the everyday realities of poor communities (Ellis 2004). While recognizing barriers to collaboration, EJ activists interested in engaging with science strongly favor a community-based participatory research (CBPR) approach (Prakash 2004).

To date, EJ organizations have varied in the degree to which they engage with science, as well as in the forms of their engagement. For example, several activists described WEACT as "unique in the movement because of its ties to science" and its commitment to creating "a strong scientific base and be[ing] able to do analysis, to not be limited to anecdotal information" (Field Notes, San Francisco 2001). EJ groups do take up science on their own terms. For example, EJ organizers in Louisiana have used relatively low-tech air-monitoring devices—"bucket brigades"—to gather evidence of pollution in communities adjacent to petrochemical facilities. This technique of doing air monitoring in fenceline communities has been taken up by EJ groups across the United States (Ottinger 2009). Whether EJ activists believe that molecular genetic research can be "taken back" by the movement defines, in large part, their orientation to these new technologies.

EJ activists have, on the whole, been skeptical of scientists' claims about the importance of research on gene-environment interaction to public health. In part, this skepticism is rooted in differences in how scientists and activists define the key obstacles to protecting and improving health. As we have seen, scientists and regulators frame the uncertainties and "bottlenecks" in toxicology testing and risk assessment and the absence of clinical intervention strategies as critical challenges in the environmental health arena. Therefore, they contend that, insofar as molecular genetics and genomics provide a means of strengthening the empirical basis for environmental regulation, streamlining and accelerating regulatory processes, and creating new treatment opportunities for people exposed to harmful substances, they will improve public health. Scientists' claims are predicated not only in confidence in science, but also in trust in the processes of environmental regulation and policy making. In contrast, environmental justice activists argue that environmental illnesses are fundamentally a consequence of how society is organized. From an EJ perspective, dimensions of race, class, and political power result in inequalities in environmental exposure and inequities in health. Further, EJ activists and their allies challenge the objectivity and neutrality of science and policy making, and they tend to be skeptical about the power of science in efforts to protect and improve the health of people of color. Therefore, EJ activists, in general, argue that improving public health and redressing health disparities require not molecular genetic and genomic technologies, but rather reorganization of the core structures of modern society. Consequently, while environmental health scientists see in molecularization a means of increasing the certainty and usability of their research, protecting their jurisdiction, and increasing the credibility of their field, most EJ activists perceive research on gene-environment interaction as a threat to their movement and its goals.

Further, EJ activists have challenged scientists and regulators to consider how molecular genetic and genomic technologies might affect members of society who are socially, politically, and economically vulnerable to environmental exposures. In contrast to other stakeholders in this arena, activists ask not *how* to address the social, ethical, and policy implications of research on gene-environment interaction, but *whether*, given these implications, such research represents the best use of public resources; often, they suggest, it does not. Likewise, in contrast to the risk assessors and regulators described in Chapter 5, environmental justice activists' responses to research on gene-environment interaction highlight the political consequences of these new techniques of measurement and the information they produce. At the same time, some EJ activists are interested in how genetic and genomic technologies could aid in their efforts to prove that environmental exposures are the cause of illnesses in specific communities.

The ways in which genetics has been used to reify and biologize racial categories, both historically and in current debates, as well as the recourse to genetics by defendants in court cases such as *Tamiko Jones, et al., v. NL Industries, et al.,* have made EJ activists especially wary of a growing role for molecular genetic research in the environmental health sciences.[15] As one activist told me, within the EJ movement, genetics has been seen as "a distraction from the issue, which is that people are being exposed and getting sick" (Field Notes, San Francisco 2001). However, "sometime around the summer of 2000," activists who were serving as advisory council members for federal research programs began to realize that "there's this genetics thing happening, and we need to figure out what it is and how it's going to impact our work" (Field Notes, New York City 2002). In February of 2002, over 350 environmental justice activists from 34 states and Puerto Rico gathered in New York City for a conference and symposium on human genetics, the environment, and communities of color (WEACT 2002).

Putting Genetics on the Agenda of the Environmental Justice Movement

The 2002 conference and symposium, Human Genetics, Environment, and Communities of Color: Ethical and Social Implications, was organized by WEACT, with sponsorship from Columbia University's Mailman School of Public Health, the NIEHS, and the EPA, as well as several private foundations. As attendees commented repeatedly throughout the two days, it was a "groundbreaking" meeting, the first national gathering addressing genetics organized by and for environmental justice activists. During the first day, activists listened to—and challenged—speakers from the environmental health sciences, medicine, law, and regulatory agencies who described genetics research and its potential implications for the future of environmental health research and policy. The second day was a symposium, attended primarily by activists, who gathered in small working groups to begin to formulate the movement's responses to genetics research and its potential implications for communities of color and the environmental justice movement.[16]

Prior to February 2002, most environmental justice activists either were not aware of molecular genetic and genomics research in the environmental health sciences or, as described above, saw it as a distraction from their core concerns. Recognizing this situation, the conference organizers sought to provide participants with both "an educational focus" and "a forum where various perspectives could be aired": "the initial idea of the conference was to educate EJ activists, primarily, about the science and about the research; what's happening, what it means, and what it has to do with our work" (Field Notes, New York 2002). Their hope was that increasing the movement's "capacity" in regard to genetics would allow activists to become actively engaged with "genetics research, and more specifically, with how it affects communities of color . . . so that we can start thinking more proactively about some of the issues" (Field Notes, WEACT 2002).[17] The organizers believed that in order to advocate for the interests of the communities they represent, environmental justice activists had to understand genetic research and its implications for governing environmental hazards: "If environmental regulations will undergo a 'revolution,' environmental justice activists will need to be at the front lines of understanding on what basis this revolution will happen" (WEACT 2002: 4). Therefore, speakers from NIEHS and the National Human Genome Research Institute (NHGRI) offered workshops on "Genetics 101" that not only covered some of the basics of genetic science (i.e., what is a gene?) but provided an overview of the NIEHS's toxicogenomics initiative. At the same time, WEACT organizers hoped that the meeting would help scientists and policy makers "get involved with" issues of environmental justice (Field Notes, WEACT 2002).

The WEACT meeting literally put genetics on the agenda of the environmental justice movement. At the closing session of the first day of the conference, one activist joked that he "now knows how to pronounce 'genome' and 'genomics'" before offering his "sincere thanks to WEACT . . . for bringing me here to get educated about these issues. We need to know about this, need to know what's going on" (Field Notes, WEACT 2002). Activists reported initially being skeptical about the conference: "Okay, we'll be honest. When we heard about this conference, we were like, 'Oh, genetics! What now?' You know?" Some said that they attended primarily out of solidarity with the organizers: "WEACT is our sister organization and we're going to support them" (Field Notes, WEACT 2002). However, during the meeting, many were convinced of the importance of the topic: "[T]o be honest, our minds were blown because the science was so accessible that we got pulled in instantly . . . we were able to see the connections to the work we're doing" (Field Notes, WEACT 2002). A movement leader commented at the close of the meeting, "Now, when I talk across the country, I'll be talking about these issues" (Field Notes, WEACT 2002). In October 2002, genetics was one of the topics for the movement's second national agenda-setting meeting, the Second National People of Color Environmental Leadership Summit.[18] As I will describe, EJ activists' "issues" in regard to genetics focus particularly on three broad concerns: (1) the molecularization of race and perceptions of responsibility for health and illness; (2) the allocation of scarce resources to research on genetics; and (3) the costs and benefits of making claims about environmental health and justice using molecular techniques.

Race and Responsibility

"Did you *see* that?" a young activist from a New York environmental justice group asked me. "It was classic!" she exclaimed. "It captured the classic dynamic of institutional power relationships. It was so symbolic. He literally turned his back to her and refused to answer her question! And everyone could see it with their own eyes!" (Field Notes, WEACT 2002). The interaction she pointed to was between Kenneth Olden, at that time the Director of the NIEHS, and Deborah Harry, the Executive Director of the Indigenous Peoples Council on Biocolonialism (IPCB).[19] The question was "how the Environmental Genome Project addresses the race issue?" It was asked during the second day of the WEACT meeting on genetics, the environment, and communities of color.

I had seen the interaction, though, perhaps unsurprisingly, I perceived it somewhat differently.[20] According to my notes, Olden responded, "I can't answer that. I don't do the race thing, because I am a scientist. Race is a social construct. I can't do anything with it"; he then stepped away from the podium (Field Notes, WEACT 2002). Olden, who grew up on a small farm in segregated Tennessee and went on to become the first African American director of a National Institute of Health, unquestionably recognizes race as a dimension of social life in America (Olden, Oral History Interview July 2004). In fact, Olden launched and supported the first environmental justice initiatives at the NIEHS during his tenure as director. Nonetheless, in this encounter, many activists perceived him as inexcusably insensitive. His comments set off what I recorded as an "explosion" of comments from activists who were outraged by their perception that he had "literally turned his back" on their concerns.

It is no coincidence that one of the most hotly contested exchanges at the WEACT conference centered on the how environmental genomics research "deals with the race issue." For many environmental justice activists, race is a primary basis of collective identity. Further, they see environmental racism as an important cause of inequalities in environmental exposures and their consequences. Therefore, from their perspective, how genetics research shapes the meaning of race and racial inequalities will be its most salient outcomes. At the WEACT conference, as well as in subsequent conversations, activists have highlighted three primary concerns about how molecular genetics and genomics will affect the meaning of race, especially in the context of environmental health and justice.

First, activists contend that research on genetic susceptibility could generate race-based data about genetic susceptibilities that could be used to usher in a new era of scientific racism. Scientists attending the WEACT meeting stated repeatedly that the goal of genetics research is to "to improve medicine, not to foster discrimination" (Field Notes, WEACT 2002). However, activists at the conference pointed to the abuses of the Tuskegee syphilis study and the "biocolonialism" of the Human Genome Diversity Project as bases for their skepticism toward scientific research on racial variations, including environmental genomic research on subpopulation variations in response to environmental exposures. Most of all, they expressed concern that research on genetic susceptibilities to environmental exposures will be used to make claims about race as a biological category. Acknowledging these concerns, a scientist attending the conference highlighted the need to be vigilant against the possibility that this research will support "racism in a new cloak." (Field Notes, WEACT 2002).

Second, and related, activists express concern about the vulnerability of communities of color to being labeled as "susceptible." As one activist at the WEACT conference stated bluntly, "I just hope that the primary outcome of all of this is not to say that some people are more susceptible than others." The NIEHS scientist to whom she addressed the question responded, "That is the outcome." However, he continued, "everyone is at risk for something, so we don't need to be so concerned . . . we'll all be identified as . . . susceptible or resistant" (Field Notes, WEACT 2002). Activists were not satisfied with this answer, which they saw as failing to recognize that "science does not exist in a social vacuum" (WEACT 2002: 6), such that communities of color are especially vulnerable to being labeled as genetically susceptible. As one activist commented in a conversation following the meeting, "I'm scared of making these arguments about people with different genetic susceptibilities, because . . . these arguments [are made] about ethnic groups. . . . You hear it all the time already and it is racist: 'those Blacks or those Hispanics have asthma because of genetics'" (Field Notes, New York 2002). Indeed, as we have seen, there is a history of such arguments being used by defendants to claim that a disease has been caused by racially specific "hereditary problems" and therefore not attributable to chemical exposures (Capek 1993).

A third danger identified by activists is that research on gene-environment interaction will divert attention from how race and class, as dimensions of social structure, shape the risk of environmental exposures and the incidence and prevalence of environmentally associated diseases. As one activist stated succinctly, "I'm concerned about science saying to Black people: 'You're sick from this exposure because you're genetically susceptible.'" Environmental justice activists argue that, even though the concept of race has no valid *biological* basis, it must be recognized as *sociopolitical* category with significant consequences for communities of color, especially in the area of environmental health. In their summary of the conference, WEACT explicitly addressed this concern, stating "the harsh realities of racism cannot be erased by a simple declaration that genetics proves that there is no such thing as race" (WEACT 2002).

The common thread running through these concerns is the issue of whether this research will "shift the perception of who is responsible for environmental health problems from *polluters* to the *individuals* living in polluted environments" (Field Notes, WEACT 2002). As this activist elaborated:

> [Say] we're struggling against the siting of the Home Depot in East Harlem. Not that this is actually happening, but this is a very plausible scenario. You hear this counter-argument, when you talk about not adding new environmental burdens to a community that has the highest asthma rate in the city and among the highest in the country . . . that this is a community comprised of people who are Puerto Rican and various Latino descents, and it's a genetic thing. *Like people there have asthma because it's in their genes and the environment is less of a factor* (Field Notes, New York 2002, emphasis added).

Related, environmental justice activists fear that genetics will shift the locus of interventions from the community to the individual level. For example, because molecular measurement techniques focus within an individual, rather than within the environment that is shared by many individuals, they may privilege individual-level approaches to environmental health and illness:

> The fear that I have with . . . genetics research . . . is shifting the perception of responsibility and the burden of responsibility back onto the individual. That's one of the reasons I'm so resistant to this concept of genetic tools. You know, the air that we breathe is a shared resource, a shared legacy, a shared human right. Also, its composition is determined by multiple external agents and factors, including people who pollute or entities that pollute. . . . So [taking measurements of the air] is a way of pinpointing . . . that responsibility for individual health is often not in the hands of the individual. The whole thing with genetics is that it goes in the opposite direction, it shifts the focus away from polluters, it shifts the focus away from sort of common and shared environment, and puts it back on the individual (Interview P01)

Put differently, environmental justice activists see genetics as potentially undermining both their diagnosis of the problem of environmental inequalities (i.e., as caused by race, class, and political disenfranchisement) and their proposed solutions, which focus on changing public policy to protect those most vulnerable to being exposed to environmental hazards.

Moreover, activists believe that genetics research could undercut their efforts to organize communities to advocate for social change. At the WEACT meeting, an activist explained that, although he was interested in genetic tools that could provide evidence of exposure, he was deeply concerned that the identification of genetic susceptibilities to environmental exposures would be used to fragment communities, undermining a key basis for mobilization, that is, a community's shared interest in reducing exposures: "What happens to the EJ community when it is partitioned into low, medium, and high risk groups?" (Field Notes, New York City 2002).[21] Activists fear also that genetic explanations could be used "as a smokescreen" (Field Notes, San Francisco 2001) to divert attention from the multiple ways that poor communities of color are vulnerable to disease. This, in turn, would weaken the moral arguments deployed by EJ activists regarding society's obligations to protect the most vulnerable of its citizens:

> . . . some of the folks living here are amongst the most vulnerable, of our
> society . . . . We are talking about people who have poor access to health
> care, people who have multiple forces of stress and few social networks to
> buffer the problems they encounter in their lives. And there is low income,
> which leads to a whole other host of challenges in life, and, you know,
> it's very difficult to have a very good diet on a budget. You go to the food
> stores here . . . you know what the grocery stores are like in central cities?
> And so there is this kind of moral obligation argument that we put for-
> ward about how the larger society does have a moral obligation to protect
> the most vulnerable, including people in our communities (Interview P01)

Consequently, many activists believe that genetics research poses a direct threat to the EJ movement. At the conclusion of the WEACT meeting, one movement leader stated his belief emphatically: "We cannot get caught in the trap of deepening the discussion about genetics and our illnesses" (Field Notes, WEACT 2002).

Allocating Resources

A second point of contention raised by activists, both at the WEACT conference and in subsequent conversations, concerns whether genetics research represents "the kind of science we need?" (Field Notes, WEACT 2002). In fact, some environmental justice activists argue that conversations about genetics and environmental health research always should start at "point zero . . . should it happen?" (Field Notes, WEACT 2002). Accordingly, these activists criticized the WEACT meeting for starting "with the assumption that genetic research would happen . . . "; according to one of the meeting organizers, "some of the Native American activists felt like this was 'participating in the evil,' to assume that the research was going to go on" (Field Notes, New York City 2002). At a meeting of the Ethical, Legal, and Social Implications Committee of the National Center for Toxicogenomics, an environmental justice activist was the only person to suggest that the committee mandate should include explicit consideration of what kinds of scientific research should be allowed to proceed with public funding (Field Notes, Washington, D.C. 2002).

Environmental justice activists argue that "science should be there to serve us," and they question the contribution of genetics research to public health. Especially in the context of limited resources for environmental health research and interventions, activists argue that priority should be given to "improving the health and quality of life for people today" by providing assistance to communities that are "living under toxic assault," rather than investing in molecular genetic and genomics technologies which may be of benefit in the future: "If the conditions that . . . people suffer from are a result of gene-environment interaction, then they are preventable by changing environmental conditions. So spending money on genetics research is misguided" (Field Notes, WEACT 2002). In recounting her experiences on a review committee at a federal agency, this activist similarly emphasized her perception of a disjuncture between genomics research and the goals of public health:

> One of the items in the research strategy was . . . something about a microarray and trying to develop a better understanding of genetic mechanisms in response to environmental factors . . . to better understand some of these molecular mechanisms. . . . But *how does that translate into improved public health?* . . . I'm sure there is a great deal of potential in

this, but . . . unless there is a clear link, especially to . . . promoting public health and preventing disease, there are other research . . . items that take priority (Field Notes, New York 2002, emphasis added)

These comments make clear also that activists do not object to allocating public funds to research, in general, but want to support research that clearly serves the end of "protect[ing] the environmental public health" (Field Notes, WEACT 2002).

Built into this critique are differences in how scientists and activists answer the question, "What is the root cause of environmental health and illness?" In a session of the WEACT meeting devoted to an introduction to research on gene-environment interaction, an activist from Communities for a Better Environment, a California-based EJ group, argued that the focus on genes and the environment should be replaced by an explicit analysis of politics and power (Field Notes, WEACT 2002). Similarly, another attendee pointed out that the "right tools for the job" of improving public health depend on what one defines as the cause of environmental illness "Genes? Or emissions, and therefore, a lax regulatory system, production and consumption . . . " (Field Notes, WEACT 2002). Activists argue, therefore, that resources would be better directed to research and interventions that would support "quality health care, safe environments with clean water and air, and surroundings that allow for and promote health behaviors" (WEACT 2002: 66).

Making Molecular Claims

Amidst these critiques, a handful of speakers at the WEACT meeting focused rather on how communities of color and EJ activists might productively use molecular genetic and genomic research to further their movement's goals. Often these speakers attempted to locate genetics research in a social justice frame. For example, several scientists contended that it was critical that communities of color not be "left out of the genomics revolution" (Field Notes, WEACT 2002). In his keynote address, Olden proposed that research on gene-environment interaction will be an integral part of reducing health disparities and creating a world "with less pain and suffering" (Field Notes, WEACT 2002; see also

Olden & White 2005). In this talk, Olden also acknowledged structural impediments to improving the health of communities of color; among the "necessary changes" he identified as important to realizing "the promise" of genome research were the elimination of disparities in access to care and the improvement of the public health infrastructure, especially at the community level (Field Notes, WEACT 2002).

Health inequalities are a central concern of EJ activists. However, in their comments at the meeting and following, activists maintained a skeptical stance toward the proposition that genetics research will improve the health of communities of color or advance the cause of social justice. Perhaps the most trenchant critique of this assertion came from Deborah Harry of the IPCB, who argued that, given that many of the diseases commonly suffered by indigenous people are "caused by economic poverty, lack of infrastructure, and contaminated environments," directing resources to genetics research, rather than to prevention and treatment, would be counterproductive (WEACT 2002: 23).

In contrast, some EJ activists expressed interest in the possibility that specific molecular genetic and genomic technologies might enable them to advance the goals of the movement, and they identified several ways that this might be accomplished. Their suggestions position genetic technologies as a means to mobilize individuals and communities to address environmental exposures and their health effects. However, as will be described, even when EJ activists are open to the possibility that molecular technologies might serve as tools for social movement mobilization, they reject scientists' claims that molecular genetic and genomic research have an important role to play in advancing public health.

First, activists suggest that molecular biomarker technologies could help to ascertain the chemical body burden of individuals living in exposed communities and measure and document the effects of those chemicals within the human body. In an interview following the meeting, an activist commented: "We would give anything if we could get an accurate sense of how much diesel a person or individual has been exposed to. . . . I like the idea of biomarkers, especially because . . . exposure assessment is so expensive and difficult" (Field Notes, Oakland 2002). Body burden testing can be done without molecular technologies.[22]

However, simply documenting the presence of chemicals in human bodies does not provide evidence of harm. In contrast, as described in Chapter 4, molecular biomarkers of effect offer the possibility of proving that exposures have had biological consequences. Thus, one activist at the WEACT conference argued, "We should focus on exposure, focus on how that changes our genes—rather than on environmental response genes" (Field Notes, WEACT 2002).

Second, and related, activists perceive body burden testing as a strategy for motivating people to mobilize around issues of environmental health and justice. As one activist stated enthusiastically in an interview: "The technology that people are excited about is body burden testing. This is the testing that people want. People are making the connections and saying 'hey, these refineries are pouring stuff into the air and I want to know what's inside of me!'" (Interview P12). Related, body burden measurements may be instrumental in generating the political will to limit environmental emissions: "It would motivate people to take action . . . knowing that they have chemicals in their bodies gets people motivated to do something" (Field Notes, Berkeley 2002; see also Altman et al. 2008). Here, EJ activists are interested in biomarkers as techniques of mobilization.

Less frequently, activists suggested that the EJ movement needed to "increase our technical capacity" in order to be able to participate effectively in legal battles in which industry may use molecular genetic information to argue against regulation (Field Notes, WEACT 2002). For example, an activist speaking at the WEACT meeting pointed out that because "the corporate community has its own toxicogenomics program" and "the agenda of companies is to decrease regulation," he "thank[ed] God that the NIEHS has the EGP and the Toxicogenomics program." He argued further that the EJ movement "should develop sufficient expertise . . . " expressing his belief that "science can address and support EJ priorities" (Field Notes, WEACT 2002). Another activist pointed out that "sometimes it takes scientific evidence to show that something's not right before anyone will believe you that it's not right" (Field Notes, San Francisco 2001). Activists also have argued that "data on genetic susceptibility should be used to set regulatory standards for general environmental health protection" (Morales 2002). In this way, activists suggest that genetic information might pose an opportunity to "raise the bar on some of our regulatory standards" (Field Notes, New York 2002).

However, even as they express interest in the specific ways that molecular technologies might be used to support the EJ movement, activists are skeptical of claims that molecular genetics and genomics can advance public health goals, independently of political change. In particular, activists express concern about the inherently post hoc focus of body burden testing and molecular biomarker technologies:

> The example . . . is lead. With children, we take a blood sample and analyze and determine how many mcg [of lead] they have in a dl of their blood, and then we issue a proclamation regarding the extent of their exposure. This is a very frightening way to assess it. You know, from a health perspective, *basically you're using a child as a monitor for lead*. By the time it has gotten to that point, it's almost too late. . . . The public health agenda needs to be intervening much earlier in the whole process of lead exposure. We can't wait until the exposures have already happened, and then treat the problem (Interview P01, emphasis added).

Consequently, she argued, "you need to be . . . wary about, about technologies that focus on after the fact assessment . . . " and emphasized the importance, rather, of preventing exposures. These comments importantly highlight the tensions between clinical interventions, which focus on exposed individuals, and public health approaches, which historically have aimed to prevent exposures from occurring.

GENES, ENVIRONMENTS, AND JUSTICE

Environmental justice activists are most inclined to see science as useful insofar as it can validate the lived experiences of people who have been exposed to environmental hazards, enabling them to prove that "we're not crazy, what we're saying is real is real" (Field Notes, San Francisco 2001). Additionally, activists see technologies that make visible otherwise undetectable exposures as having the potential to motivate people to mobilize against environmental injustice. Under such conditions, EJ activists will engage with scientific technologies. As an EPA scientist (and former activist) reflected, "when community groups want to learn something, they learn it. If they want to do gas chromatography studies and you give them the machine, they'll learn how to use it, maintain it, do research, do really good work with it" (Field Notes, San Francisco 2001; see also Corburn 2005). Simply put, when activists can deploy scientific technologies to advance movement goals, they often will do so.

However, EJ activists reject the claim of environmental health scientists that genomics is the key to improving the public's health. From the perspective of many EJ activists, these claims lack empirical credibility; they simply do not fit with activists' experience of the world. Activists are particularly suspicious of the claim that molecular research will promote public health by refining the regulatory process; they argue rather that "laws and regulations do not equal protection, they are too often undermined" (Field Notes, WEACT 2002). Further, they see genomic approaches as unable to accommodate the questions that, from an environmental justice perspective, are central to public health in the United States: "questions about how we organize ourselves as a society, questions about corporate accountability, social and environmental justice, questions about who bears the burden of industrial society? . . . questions about what is progress, what is technology and when do we stop? When is it enough?" (Field Notes, Oakland 2001). Moreover, activists reject scientists' visions of the potential biomedical applications of molecular genetic technologies, arguing that interventions "after the fact" of exposure are insufficient; rather, they contend, the goal must be preventing harmful exposures in the first place. Put simply, on the whole, activists are critical of proposed applications of molecular genetics in the environmental health sciences.

Environmental health scientists are enthusiastic about the potential of molecular genetic and genomic technologies to "bring the human back in" to environmental health research (Field Notes, NIEHS 2002). As described in Chapter 4, molecular epidemiology has enabled scientists to refocus their research inside human bodies, overturning the environmental health sciences' long-standing reliance on using animal models to assess the effects of environmental chemicals. However, as EJ activists' critiques make clear, translating from the "thin" representations of humans in the laboratory—where molecular biomarkers and cDNA microarrays provide measures of human bodies and their vital capacities—to the complex and unequal settings where people live, work, and play poses a profound challenge to the environmental health sciences.

Specifically, thinking of health and illness as products of gene-environment interaction requires that the environment be conceptualized and measured as something that interacts with genes. Developing models that span from "cells to society" or from "neurons to neighborhoods" is a focus of contemporary research in both the social and the life sciences.[23] These efforts may lead to ways of measuring gene-environment interaction that include, rather than obfuscate, aspects of social and political inequalities. However, in the meanwhile, many scientists continue to conceptualize race as a biological construct, rather than as a social and political reality (Epstein 2007; Fullwiley 2007; Shim 2005). The critiques and concerns of environmental justice activists thus call attention precisely to the aspects of human life that are most likely to become invisible when the environment is conceptualized at the molecular level. Of particular concern in the context of environmental research, these include dimensions of social structure—such as race and class—that are strongly correlated with the risk of exposure to environmental hazards (Brulle & Pellow 2006; Evans & Kantrowitz 2002).

As a means of addressing these concerns, some EJ activists argue for a community-based participatory research approach to environmental health science in general and to research on gene-environment interaction in particular. Among the recommendations that emerged from the WEACT symposium in 2002 are incorporating community oversight and agenda setting in genetics research in the environmental health sciences and building truly egalitarian and ongoing partnerships between scientists and communities of color. The goal, according to EJ activists, must be a "transparent, collaborative approach" that will "maximiz[e] promised benefits" of molecular genetic research within traditionally disenfranchised communities (Sze & Prakash 2004: 744).

The San Francisco Department of Public Health offers an intriguing example of how community engagement can broaden the scope of environmental health concerns. There, public health officials have decided to expand their environmental health mandate to include issues such as crime, housing, and food access (Corburn 2009). The Department of Public Health made this decision in response to a community survey in Bay View Hunter's Point (BVHP), which revealed that "residents' priority 'environmental health concerns' were crime, unemployment, [lack of] access to healthy food, and housing conditions" (Corburn 2009: 105). The focus of the BVHP residents on these broader social issues was perhaps all the more powerful given that BVHP is burdened with myriad chemical hazards, including a Superfund site (a former naval shipyard and repair facility), leaking underground fuel tanks, a Pacific Gas and Electric power plant, and numerous small industries (Corburn 2009: 103–104). BHVP residents have been advocating around issues of environmental health and justice since the early 1990s, focusing especially on the community's high rates of asthma and cancer. Simply put, this community is well aware of the existence of chemical exposures and their potential consequences. Nonetheless, residents of BVHP articulate a conceptualization of the environment that goes beyond chemical pollutants to include social and economic factors.

Despite such initiatives, there are significant institutional barriers to including social, economic, and political factors in environmental health research. To begin, both the style of thought of environmental health scientists and, related, their orientation to contributing to environmental health risk assessment, regulation, and policy making mitigate against defining the environment in gene-environment interaction in terms of social, political, or economic contexts. In general, conceptualizing the environment at multiple levels—"from cells to society"—is not well accommodated by the methodological reductionism of the life sciences (Sloan 2000) or the structure of academic fields. Additionally, as described in Chapter 5, the research that scientists undertake to inform risk assessment and regulation in the U.S. examines how a single chemical is likely to affect the health of a "standard human." The environment of the environmental health research, therefore, is often conceptualized, measured, and assessed one chemical at a time.

However, the increasing focus of scientists and policy makers on health disparities in the United States is generating both new institutional spaces and resources for integrating measures of the social environment into molecular genetic and genomic research (IOM 2006). It has also led to increasing recognition of the need to engage directly with people from communities disproportionately burdened with poor health outcomes (Corburn 2009). As this EJ activist suggested, "the problem" with the environmental health sciences is that " . . . there is no integration across the research on social and economic factors, like environmental justice, and science . . . [the] group working on socioeconomic status and environmental health . . . is totally unrelated to the biological and biochemical work being done" (Field Notes, San Francisco 2001). If so, then some promise may be found in new forms of research that seek to assess the biological consequences of both social structures and environmental exposures. Again, however, molecularization is having powerful effects, as described in the concluding chapter.

Conclusion

The jumping off place for this analysis was a puzzle: The defining mission, as well as the professional jurisdiction, of the environmental health sciences is to understand how environmental exposures affect human health. Yet, over the past thirty years, many of these scientists have shifted the focus of their research away from the external, ambient environment to look deep inside the human body, at the molecular level—a shift that has consequences not only for how scientists do their work, but also for how we, as a society, understand and seek to control the potentially harmful effects of environmental exposures. What accounts for this transformation? And how do we understand its consequences? What aspects of risk become more and less visible when the environment conceptualized and operationalized at the molecular level?

Explanations of transformations in scientific practices tend to focus on technologically determinist narratives, on "bandwagons," or on actor-network accounts. In the first case, the rise of gene-environment interaction is explained straightforwardly as a consequence of powerful new technologies. This is a narrative favored by many of the scientists whom I interviewed; they frequently described themselves as being carried along on a "roller coaster" or "tsunami" of new forms of data. In the latter two, transformation is explained as a consequence of the emergence of a shared commitment to using particular tools to articulate and solve specific scientific problems. This form of explanation is favored by symbolic interactionist analyses of changes in scientific practice, such as the rise of genetics in cancer research (Fujimura 1996). It is also the underlying logic of actor-network theory's emphasis on "the operations that link technical devices, statements, and human beings" into networks of inter-related and interdependent roles (Callon 1995: 50; see also Latour 1987). Although these explanations do not preclude analyses of scientific fields or institutions, their focus tends to be on social relationships between individuals and laboratories, rather than on structural relationships between individuals, institutions, and broader social, economic, and cultural domains (Bottero & Crossley 2011).[1]

My account diverges from these explanations. I contend that environmental health scientists turned to molecular genetic research to solve problems of power that are central to their field and its institutions: scientific authority, institutional jurisdiction, and access to valued resources, both financial and symbolic. To be sure, these problems often first appear in scientists' narratives as methodological or technical challenges. And, undoubtedly, solving these problems requires coordinated action among individuals and institutions. However, both scientists' perceived need to address such challenges and the strategies that appear to offer acceptable solutions are shaped both by the field and the arena in which it is embedded. Simply put, research on gene-environment interaction has been compelling to environmental health scientists not only because it provides a new set of techniques for coordinating their investigations into the health effects of environmental exposures. Rather, research on gene-environment interaction is compelling to environmental health scientists insofar as it promises a diverse array of strategies for redressing the field's structural vulnerabilities.

The structural vulnerabilities of the environmental health sciences derive from the field's central research foci, relationships to other fields, social identity, and exposure to a contentious political arena. To begin, in contrast to biomedical research, the environmental health sciences are defined by their focus on preventing disease, primarily by serving as an empirical basis for public policy. Focusing on prevention at the population level has given environmental health scientists a way to distinguish their research and its applications from biomedicine, with its mission of providing clinical treatment to individuals. However, these foci produce two of the most profound challenges to the field. First, as a consequence of its ties to risk assessment, regulation, and associated legal contests, a wide variety of stakeholders—including regulated industries, consumer protection advocates, and environmental health and justice activists representing exposed communities—regularly contest both the methods and the findings of environmental health science. Insofar as scientific authority is based on the ability to contain and isolate disputes from general scrutiny (Collins 1985; Shapin 1994; Panofsky 2011), the authority of the environmental health sciences is enduringly precarious. Contestations from regulated industries, in particular, have shaped research practices in the environmental health sciences, motivating an unending quest to increase "certainty," especially of toxicological research. Meanwhile, environmental health scientists work with a constant awareness that research finding harmful effects will be met with procedural, empirical, and, if it leads to regulation, legal challenges. A toxicologist described the NTP as a "catalyst" for research in the field precisely because its evaluations of chemicals serve as a "the engine . . . for an awful lot of research, especially that carried out by industry to refute the findings" (Interview S38). In the words of a cancer epidemiologist: "It's like an ongoing cold war. . . . We find that a chemical has a carcinogenic effect. Industry does its own study. We have to respond to their findings" (Field Notes, Bethesda 2011). Indeed, the regulatory agencies must respond to industry's studies even when they are obviously flawed; in the words of a former OSHA official, this has become "a part of the game" (Michaels 2008: 55).

At the same time, environmental health scientists' focus on disease prevention via public policy constrains both the available funding and the markets for their research. In recent years, some environmental health scientists have endeavored to establish a "more biomedical" approach to environmental health and illness, which would encompass clinical interventions for exposed or at-risk individuals.[2] Still, as we have seen, policy makers are quick to hold the environmental health sciences accountable to their public health mandate (US GPO 2007).[3] Moreover, many environmental health scientists are deeply committed to the traditional orientation of their field toward disease prevention via public policy, identifying strongly as public servants. Insofar as environmental health research does not orient to biomedical interventions but rather to broad policy or behavioral interventions, the federal government will continue to be the most important funder of environmental health science in the United States. As such, both formal institutional arrangements and scientists' identities support the continued connections between environmental health science and risk assessment and regulation. This, in turn, ensures that it will be exposed to ongoing challenge and contestation by powerful—and, in the case of industry, well funded—stakeholders in the environmental health arena.

At the turn of the twenty-first century, environmental health scientists faced two additional challenges that made molecular tools compelling: (1) the ascendance of genetic understandings of human health and illness and (2) the perception that their field needed to strengthen the certainty and legitimacy of their research, both to meet the standards of their scientific peers and to make it more robust to challenge by outside parties. First, in the years leading up to the mapping of the human genome, many scientists and members of the public held great hope that the Human Genome Project would unlock the secrets of human health, illness, and identity. James Watson, the first director of the HGP, exemplified such expectations when he pronounced, "We used to think our fate was in the stars. Now we know, in large measure, our fate is in our genes" (quoted by Jaroff 1989). In 1988, National Research Council (NRC) report argued that sequencing the human genome would "allow rapid progress to occur in the diagnosis and ultimate control of many human diseases" (in Green et al. 2011: 211). In his tireless advocacy for the HGP, Francis Collins, then Director of the NHGRI, proclaimed that "it is hard to imagine that genomic science will not soon reveal the mysteries of hereditary factors in heart disease, cancer, diabetes, mental illness, and a host of other conditions" (2001: 643). These pronouncements raised profound concerns among environmental health scientists about whether a genocentric view of human bodies and lives would lead scientists, policy makers, and the public to ignore, minimize, or discount entirely the role of environmental exposures in creating human health and illness.[4]

Second, and related, environmental health scientists—and the scientific advisory boards that guide the development of priorities and practices of environmental health research at institutions such as the NIEHS and EPA—were concerned that specific subfields and institutions of environmental health research were in dire danger of losing status, funding, and political support. Most often, scientists expressed these concerns in relation to a perception that the methods of environmental health research were "falling behind" the leading edge of life sciences research—an edge defined, at that time, by genomic technologies that examined biological processes deep inside the body, at the molecular level.

Advocates for molecular genetic approaches to environmental health research framed the rise of genetics—as well as the specter of the demise of their central institutions—as both a threat and an opportunity for the environmental health sciences.[5] We can see this framing strategy especially in the strong rationale for molecularization offered in the consensus critique. Most broadly, a consensus critique is a strategy for bringing together stakeholders with substantive political, economic, and/or social differences by emphasizing a set of narrowly defined shared concerns. Social actors central to the construction of a consensus critique often position themselves as neutral in regard to the substantive outcomes that will result from addressing these concerns; they focus, rather, on improvements to a process that actors in the field cannot easily contest, such as increasing efficiency or accuracy, and their contributions to the field as a whole. In this particular case, the consensus critique has centered on the ways that genomic technologies could improve the *process* of toxicology testing and risk assessment. It emphasizes especially how focusing inside human bodies and at the molecular level will decrease the uncertainties inherent in current techniques, which rely on extrapolation from highly standardized animal models exposed to high doses of a single chemical to diverse human populations encountering myriad exposures in their daily lives. By promising a means of doing toxicology testing and risk assessment that would be faster, less expensive, and more certain—while remaining determinedly agnostic about the consequences of such changes on the outcomes of regulatory decision making—the consensus critique has facilitated support for the development of molecular techniques from actors with strongly divergent political and economic interests. This support is manifest in the emergence of collaborations such as Tox21, which seek to establish a new, molecular basis for environmental health risk assessment and regulation.

At the same time, the ascendance of gene-environment interaction in the environmental health sciences has been facilitated by the interpretive flexibility that it offers to scientists; there is room under the banner of gene-environment interaction for a wide variety of practices. These include both older lines of inquiry in environmental health research—such as environmental mutagenesis and carcinogenesis—and new, hybrid subfields—such as environmental genomics, molecular epidemiology, and toxicogenomics. Most broadly, this interpretive flexibility means that gene-environment interaction refers both to research that examines how genes and gene expression are affected by environmental exposures and research that centers on how human genetic susceptibility makes some people relatively more vulnerable to the harmful effects of environmental chemicals. Groups with divergent interests, then, have been able to align themselves with the overarching project of molecularizing environmental health research.

By encompassing these varied research foci, gene-environment interaction also has made space for a diverse array of possible interventions, with varied biopolitical consequences. Again, under this same banner, we see both initiatives such as Tox21, focused on the molecularization of the risk assessment process, and the efforts of molecular epidemiologists to develop clinical interventions targeting individuals who may be at higher risk of illness following an environmental exposure. This latter approach highlights the potential of molecularization to move the environmental health sciences closer to the "dominant epidemiological framework" (Brown 2007), with its emphasis on individual, behavioral risk factors and effacement of the social structural determinants of environmental exposures and illness. Simply put, molecular measurements— which locate genetic susceptibilities, environmental exposures, and their effects inside the human body—individualize the risks of exposures most often experienced in settings shared by multiple individuals, such as neighborhoods, workplaces, schools, and playgrounds. Individualization, in turn, supports clinical approaches to problems heretofore addressed via public policy. As one researcher imagines, "These are things that you could eventually see in a doctor's office . . . it wouldn't take too great a stretch of the imagination to expect physicians to regularly screen patients for 100 or so of the most implicated chemicals to assess disease risk"; in this way, environmental health and illness are aligned with "the vision of the future of medicine being more predictive and more personalized" (Harmon 2010: 2). This approach may well benefit individuals who are exposed to harmful chemicals in the environment. However, as EJ activists suggest, rather than monitoring and treating individuals exposed to environmental health risks, the logic of primary prevention would dictate that we redouble efforts to prevent exposures from occurring in the first place.

Thus, although diverse forms of molecularization—and the further scientization of environmental health risk assessment and regulation— may promise remedies to the structural vulnerabilities of the environmental health sciences, they also introduce new domains of contention in the environmental health arena. We know far too little about how industry will respond to the emergence of molecularized regulatory science.[6] Nonetheless, we can see the effects of scientists' anticipation of how industry will respond, especially in their efforts to demonstrate the relevance and reliability of genomic technologies, such as microarrays in toxicology testing. These efforts are a conscious response to the requirements for validating alternative testing methods; at the same time, they prepare new forms of science for challenges under the *Daubert* test, which governs the admissibility of scientific evidence in the courts

(Jasanoff 2005; Michaels 2008). That is to say, environmental health scientists clearly anticipate challenges from regulated industries, and their efforts to prepare for these challenges is shaping the emergence of new knowledge and practices in this field.

EJ activists allege that these strategies run the risk of reinforcing biological conceptualizations of race, diverting critical resources from efforts to identify and ameliorate harmful exposures, and obscuring the social, political, and economic factors that make people of color and of lower socioeconomic status more likely to be exposed to a variety of toxic substances. Consequently, although some EJ activists have expressed limited interest in the potential of molecular techniques to improve their ability to substantiate their claims, on the whole, EJ activists remain critical of the increasing focus on gene-environment interaction within the environmental health sciences. Their critiques point to the social, political, and economic issues that are sidelined in the agenda set by the consensus critique. They also highlight the importance of questions about what the environment *is*, when conceptualized and operationalized at the molecular level, and what aspects of risk thereby become more and less visible.

In these final pages, I examine some intended and unintended consequences of the continued ascendance of gene-environment interaction in the environmental health sciences. This account provides an update on aspects of research on gene-environment interaction that have emerged since 2005, when I concluded my fieldwork; at the same time, it highlights the ongoing salience of the themes elaborated in the preceding pages. To begin, I contend that gene-environment interaction has opened up a space for research on the environment across the life sciences. Moreover, the kinds of environments considered in this research have been expanding dramatically, now routinely including specific measures of the social environment. However, environmental exposures—whether chemical or social—are pervasively molecularized in this research. This turn of events highlights the importance of molecularization as an analytic concept. Put differently, if following the lead of the geneticization thesis, if we asked only whether scientists have continued to study environmental causes of variation in human health and social outcomes, we would miss the opportunity to observe profound changes in how the environment is conceptualized and operationalized in this research. Second, I suggest that addressing the structural vulnerabilities of the environmental health sciences will require thinking beyond the limitations elucidated in the consensus critique. The chapter concludes with a consideration of the implications of this analysis for both sociology and the environmental health sciences.

THE PLACE OF THE ENVIRONMENT

In contrast to the predictions of the geneticization thesis, the genomic revolution has not resulted in an effacement of the environment in research on human health and illness. In fact, as noted by researchers across the life sciences and social sciences, genomics has had the paradoxical effect of calling attention to the importance of social and environmental factors vis-à-vis human health and illness (Olden & White 2005; Pescosolido 2006; Schwartz & Collins 2007). Speaking at a meeting of population health researchers in 2009, a prominent science policy maker noted, "The leading edge of population health is the most reductionist endeavor at NIH—the Human Genome Project—*because it actually highlights the importance of social and environmental determinants*" (Author's Notes, 2009). High-profile genomics researchers now aver that the "huge amounts of exuberance and enthusiasm" about the completion of the HGP led to the "overstating" of the immediate promise of genomics (Green, in Kaiser 2011: 660). Likewise, they now speak of a need to be "a little bit more realistic and a little more cautious" in their predictions about when and how genomics research will begin its long predicted transformation of the practice of biomedicine (Green, in Kaiser 2011: 660). In fact, in a paper in the prestigious journal *Nature* marking the ten-year anniversary of the draft sequence of the human genome, the leaders of NHGRI, writing on behalf of the Institute, stated bluntly that "profound improvements in the effectiveness of healthcare cannot realistically be expected for many years" (Green et al. 2011: 204). According to genome scientists, there is now widespread recognition that the complexity of the human genome *and its interactions with the environment* mean that identifying how genes "interact with environmental factors" will be an important part of "translating genome based knowledge into health benefits" (Collins et al. 2003: 840). As science and technology studies (STS) scholars have noted: "It is almost ironic that the deeper biologists delve into the human body and the more fine-grained and molecularised their analyses of the body become, the less they are able to ignore the many ties that link the individual body and its molecules to the spatio-temporal contexts within which it dwells" (Niewohner 2011: 290).

Indeed, soon after the completion of the HGP in 2003, the leadership of the NHGRI had begun making statements about the importance of understanding of gene-environment interactions. In a 2003 paper entitled "Welcome to the Genomics Era," Guttmacher and Collins noted that it "bears repeating" that "even in the genomic era, it is not genes alone but *the interplay of genetic and environmental factors* that determines phenotype (i.e., health or disease)" (2003: 997, emphasis added). To better understand this interplay, the NHGRI convened a Gene Environment Interplay Workshop in 2010. This meeting brought together one hundred fifty scientists, representing a wide array of fields, to evaluate the state of the science in the study of gene-environment interactions in complex disease and to make recommendations regarding research priorities, challenges, and next steps (Bookman et al. 2011). The participants at the workshop called for an integrative model of complex disease, emphasizing particularly the need to bring measures of environmental exposures into biomedical research. Today, the leadership of the NHGRI also advocates for the "integration" of genomic information with environmental exposure in order to generate "a much fuller understanding of disease aetiology" (Green et al. 2011: 208).

Concern about health disparities in the United States (Williams 2005) also has motivated a focus on social and environmental conditions. In 2011, a request for information to guide strategic planning at the CDC's Office of Public Health Genomics revealed public expectations that genomics serve the goal of reducing health disparities.[7] In recent publications, leading genomics scientists have noted particularly that integrating environmental measures and interventions into biomedical research will be critical to efforts to remediate health disparities in the United States. For example, writing in *Nature*, Green and colleagues observed, "Most documented causes of health disparities are not genetic, but are due to poor living conditions and limited access to healthcare" (Green et al. 2011: 210).[8]

With the emergence of gene-environment interaction as a focus of research across the life sciences, scientists have begun to call for better measurements of environmental exposures and for the inclusion of exposure data in large databases, including, but not limited to, those being used in genomics research (Rappaport & Smith 2010; Schwartz & Collins 2006; Wild 2005). These calls often emphasize that understanding common, complex diseases requires "that both environmental exposures and genetic variation be reliably measured" (Wild 2005: 1847); however, to date, the disproportionate investment in measuring genetic risk factors means that researchers often use cutting-edge genomics technologies to assess genetic variation and gene expression, while using questionnaires to characterize environmental exposures (Rappaport & Smith 2010: 460). Environmental health researchers have suggested that better measurements of environmental exposures may clarify associations between genetic variations and diseases that "currently seem completely random" (Harmon 2010: 3). Similarly, some scientists have suggested that the inadequacy of extant measurement techniques for capturing the complexity of the environment may explain the ongoing challenge of replicating results from genomic studies and the limited results produced by many genome-wide association studies (GWAS) (MacArthur 2008; Patel, Bhattacharya, & Butte 2010). There have also been calls for the broader dissemination of information, to policy makers and the public, about disparities in social and environmental determinants of health. For example, in 2011, an Institute of Medicine (IOM) committee recommended that "the Department of Health and Human Services produce an annual report to inform all policy-makers, all health-system sectors, and the public about important trends and disparities in social and environmental determinants that affect health" (2011: 6).

Privately, environmental health scientists muse about whether genomics researchers really believe that the environment is "is as big a player as it is" and, related, whether the leaders of NHGRI have fully "yet internalized" their view that "you've got to have that environmental trigger and without it nothing's going to happen" (Field Notes, NIEHS 2004). Funding for genomics continues to outpace funding for research on environmental exposures; even in the collaborative Genes, Environment, and Health Initiative (GEI), which endeavors to find "the genetic and environmental roots of common diseases," nearly twice as much funding is allocated for the "genes" component of the project. [9]

Nonetheless, some major initiatives seek to make it easier for genomics researchers to measure the environment in gene-environment interaction. For example, the PhenX Project, funded by NHGRI, aims to facilitate the integration of genomics and epidemiological research, primarily by providing genomics researchers with "high-quality, relatively low-burden measures" of environments, human behaviors, and phenotypes.[10] These measures are made available online, free of cost, in a Tool Kit, which provides researchers with detailed protocols for collecting the measures, as well as documentation of their development and validation. PhenX has not yet made data available regarding the uptake of the Tool Kit or its use in specific studies. The website does provide information about the most frequently viewed research domains, which, as of May 2011, included the domain containing measures of environmental exposures.[11]

Moreover, new research practices are already emerging from those described here, taking as their focus what has been called the human *exposome* or the *envirome*. First proposed by a molecular epidemiologist, the intention behind exposome research is to serve as a "bridge" between molecular biomarker research and genomics technologies in order to characterize "life course environmental exposures (including lifestyle factors) from the prenatal period onward" (Wild 2005: 1848). This approach would require profound changes in the conduct of environmental health research. First, advocates of exposomics contend that environmental health science has been limited by its "parochial" division of exposures into categories such as air and water pollution, occupation, diet and physical activity, stress, and so on (Rappaport & Smith 2010). Therefore, they propose a reconceptualization of environmental exposures that is not bound by these categories but rather encompasses a wide variety of external and internal factors relevant to human biological processes and their effects.[12] Second, exposome research focuses wholly within the human body. The environment of concern in exposomics is "the body's internal chemical environment"; the term *exposures* refers to "the amounts of biologically active chemicals in this internal environment" (Rappaport & Smith 2010: 460). This includes not only toxicants that have entered the body from chemicals in air, water, and food, but also chemicals produced by the body as a consequence of inflammation, infection, gut flora, and other internal processes (Rappaport & Smith 2010). Third, and related, exposome research replaces the hypothesis-driven model of the environmental health sciences, with its focus on the associations between individual chemicals and diseases, with the "global analysis" and hypothesis-generating approach used in genomics in order to "allow the biologic system to tell you what's really important" (Arnaud 2010: 2).[13] With its focus on human bodies living in complex social and physical environments, exposomics offers a new way of studying the effects of environmental exposures. However, like other molecular techniques, it locates the scientific gaze wholly within the human body. This raises questions about the capacity of exposomics to encompass the social, political, and economic conditions that put people at risk of risk[14] (Link & Phelan 1995).

Under the banner of enviromics, scientists have begun to conduct environment-wide association studies (EWAS) that follow the protocols developed by GWAS to comprehensively consider the environmental factors that play a role in the etiology of common complex diseases, such as diabetes, cardiovascular disease, and cancer. In a study that serves as a prototype for EWAS research, researchers found associations between environment exposures and Type 2 diabetes with effect sizes "comparable to the highest odds ratios seen in GWAS" (Patel, Bhattacharya, & Butte 2010: 8). In their conclusions, the researcher advocated for approaches to analysis, such as EWAS, which can be conducted in a "non-selective" fashion, that is, which provide a means of learning about how multiple environmental factors influence disease.[15]

Viewed from the analytic perspective developed in this book, what is remarkable about both exposome and envirome research is their potential to unhinge environmental health science from the regulatory imperative—to provide toxicological assessments of single agents— and the methodological challenges and associated uncertainties that form the core of the consensus critique. Moreover, they represent an -omics approach to environmental health research that transcends the hypothesis testing model of the traditional life sciences. While potentially threatening the substantive division of labor in epidemiology, these new approaches maintain the field's commitment to doing research that is deeply relevant to public health and public policy. Their emergence points to the possibility that the processes of molecularization described in this book may have profound, if wholly unintended, consequences. As has happened in the past, looking inside the human body—and, in this case, at the molecular level—might force a confrontation with new questions about the ways in which environmental exposures shape human health and illness (Sellers 1997).

Even more broadly, there is now pervasive interest in one form of gene-environment interaction—epigenetics—across the life sciences and, increasingly, within the social sciences as well. Scientists contend that epigenetics offers a more complex way of understanding how the environment shapes human health and illness, especially by examining early life exposures that may contribute to the risk for adult onset diseases (Olden et al. 2011). At a strategic planning stakeholder workshop held at the NIEHS in 2011, participants emphasized the importance of epigenetics, voting to establish "understanding how early life environmental exposures impact development and health across the life span" as their top research priority.[16] The life course perspective embedded in epigenetics also greatly expands the kinds of environments seen as relevant to human development and the hypothesized power of the "health-determining" effects of those environments (Landecker 2011: 189).

Epigenetics, like research on gene-environment interaction more broadly, tends to use molecular measurements to operationalize the environments in which bodies are embedded. This again highlights the limitations of the geneticization thesis; that is, even when the environment retains explanatory power in etiologies of human health and illness, it may be pervasively transformed. Further, such conceptual and operational transformations in scientific research may have profound biopolitical implications; they shape the kinds of biomedical and public policy interventions that seem efficacious, reasonable, and desirable. Thus, we are brought back to the question: "What is the environment in research on gene-environment interactions?"

Molecular Environments

What does it mean to conceptualize the environment at the molecular level? How do scientists operationalize lifestyle or poverty when seeking to ascertain the effects of social environments on gene expression? The salience of these questions is heightened by the ongoing efforts of environmental health scientists to *expand* the definition of the environment to include not only physical and chemical exposures, but also "your lifestyle choice . . . diet, nutrition, certain pharmaceutical exposures, and things like poverty" (Olden, Oral History Interview July 2004). The NIEHS' advocacy for this broader definition, which includes "the toxicant environment, and the built environment, the natural environment, the social environment" (Interview S27), began at much the same time as efforts to molecularize environmental health research. Initially, I saw this as a paradoxical set of events and asked the scientists I interviewed to help me understand how they would scale up to social structure and scale down to molecules simultaneously. In recent years, epigenetics researchers have developed two main kinds of strategies for meeting these challenges in laboratory settings.

In the first strategy, scientists choose a single chemical exposure that stands in for the environment in the dyad of gene-environment interaction. For example, Landecker describes how food and, more particularly, the bioactive molecules of foods become formalized as an "environmental exposure" in epigenetics research. The experimental formalization of food as environment effectively "proposes a specific molecular route from inside to outside, and suggests a mechanism by which the wars and famines and abundant harvests of one generation can affect the metabolic systems of another" (Landecker 2011: 178). This form of molecularization has paradoxical effects. On the one hand, it offers a means of

conceptualizing how socioeconomic differences—as manifest in differences in sociomaterial environments—become embedded biologically.[17]
On the other, it renders not only those very socioeconomic differences,
but also the food itself, as a "fuzzy background" for the bioactive molecules that emerge as the real actors shaping human bodies and their
vulnerabilities (Landecker 2011: 184). Likewise, research that centers on
individual environmental chemicals and their interactions with human
genetic material generally does not attend to the socially determined
processes through which exposure occurs.

A second strategy relies on the formalization of complex social environments via animal studies. For example, epigenetics researchers interested in the relationship between socioeconomic position[18] and health
might investigate what they conceptualize as "early life adversity" by
limiting rat pups' time with their mother or by reducing the bedding
and nesting material available in a cage (Niewohner 2011: 289). Thus,
the messiness of complex environmental contexts and dynamics of social change are made amenable to the demands of laboratory research;
they are standardized in ways that enable their statistical correlation
with changes in the materiality of bodies (Niewohner 2011: 289). This
approach is rooted in models of human health and illness that theorize
chronic stress as a major cause of health disparities in the United States
(House 2002; Williams & Mohammed 2009). In place of the question,
"How does stress get under the skin?" epigenetics researchers ask how
the environment—including the social environment—gets under the
skin (Olden et al. 2011). What remains to be seen is whether focusing on
the effects of social environment inside the human body and at the molecular level highlights or makes even more "fuzzy" the social, political,
and economic causes of these effects.[19]

We thus return to the concept of *biopolitics*, which calls attention to
all the conditions under which humans live, procreate, maintain or lose
their health, and die (Foucault 1978/1990; Dean 1999: 99). Empirical analysis of molecularization highlights how the objects conceptualized and
operationalized in this biopolitical paradigm may be linked to—or may
obscure—broader social, political, and economic conditions. Such linkages have clear implications for the efforts of individuals and institutions

to understand and intervene in the health not only of individuals but of populations.

ALTERNATIVE PATHWAYS[20]

Sociologists have rendered compelling critiques of the dominant epidemiological paradigm, suggesting that the environmental health sciences offer a more promising approach to understanding the effects of toxic exposures (Brown 2007). Likewise, activists have called for increased funding for environmental health research focused on disease etiology, in contrast to biomedical research that takes disease incidence for granted and focuses rather on treatment. My analysis suggests that the very features of the environmental health sciences that appeal to these constituencies—its orientation to primary prevention via public policy and its jurisdictional focus on the ambient environment—have made the field structurally vulnerable. Consequently, as part of efforts to strengthen the credibility and certainty of their science, many environmental health scientists seek to align their research practices and products with the dominant epidemiological paradigm, with its focus on individual-level disease risk factors and on prevention and treatment strategies. I conclude this book by considering the implications of this analysis, both for sociology and environmental health science.

Structural Vulnerabilities and Exposed Scientific Fields

This analysis has clear implications for how sociologists study the transformation of scientific practices, including but not limited to the transformations wrought by molecularization. Although my work has focused on the rise of gene-environment interaction in the environmental health sciences, it highlights, more broadly, the importance of analyzing the ties between fields and the political and economic arenas in which scientific fields are located.[21] In contrast to research that focuses on the internal workings of fields, "depicting them as largely self-contained, autonomous worlds," this case joins with other recent work that points to the critical role of "extrafield relationships" (Hess 2011: 334), "broader field environments" (Fligstein & McAdam 2012) or arenas (Clarke 1998; Jasper 2004) in which fields are embedded. Not only do threats and opportunities arise from connected fields (Fligstein &McAdam 2012: 169), but the very structure of a field, its strengths and vulnerabilities, and its capacity for accommodating contention are all shaped by its relationships to other fields. Simply put, in order to understand stability and change in science, one must assess the relative autonomy of a scientific field, the nature of its ties and exposures to other fields, and how these change over time.[22]

For example, I have argued that the ties between the field of the environmental health sciences and the process of risk assessment and regulation have shaped the terms of contention and debate about what good environmental health science is.[23] Consequently, knowledge production in the environmental health sciences—and its institutions—is deeply shaped by the arena in which it is located. Not only are scientific claims and the political struggle for scientific authority impossible to separate (Lave 2012); in this case, scientific claims, the political struggle for scientific authority, and the ongoing controversies and contestations that are inextricably linked to environmental politics have become deeply intertwined. [24] This suggests that we must more explicitly consider how both historical and ongoing political controversies and market forces shape what is seen as good or valuable scientific knowledge in specific fields.[25] At issue here is not whether government, industry, and advocacy-based science is accurate or biased, but rather how political and economic forces condition the emergence of specific research agendas in the sciences.[26]

This analysis thereby gives rise to new, exciting, and challenging questions, such as: Why are some fields more successful than others in limiting their exposure to the political and/or economic dynamics of the arenas in which they are located? Does a field's exposure to political or economic pressures tend to change over time (i.e., at different stages of its development)? If so, why or how does it change? What are more and less successful strategies for limiting exposure? What are the scope conditions for such successes? Finally, how do strategies for limiting the vulnerabilities created by such exposures shape what we know—and do not know—about the world we live in? Understanding these dynamics will require empirical social scientific research that compares fields to each other and examines field dynamics over time.

To be clear, my intention is not to suggest that our understanding of emergent forms of science can or should be reduced to political or economic stakes; nor is this to merely recapitulate the argument that science is politics by other means. Rather, I contend that political and economic interests have played an underacknowledged role in determining the emergence of new forms of knowledge production by creating structural vulnerabilities in scientific fields that scientists are compelled to redress. These dynamics have deep and lasting consequences for our world and our visions of possible futures.

Beyond Consensus

One of the central arguments of this book is that environmental health scientists' efforts to address the structural vulnerabilities of their field have profound consequences for what we know—and what we do not know—about the somatic vulnerabilities of our bodies. Put differently, how environmental health scientists understand the vulnerabilities of their field has played an important role in determining their interest in emergent forms of knowledge production.

These dynamics may be most easily seen in the consensus critique that has been so central to the molecularization of the environmental health sciences. The consensus critique is a powerful and strategically skillful articulation of the vulnerabilities of the environmental health sciences in the context of risk assessment and regulation. It has been a powerful narrative both in mobilizing support for novel techniques and in facilitating the development of new networks and collaborations in the environmental health sciences; both have been essential to the emergence of research on gene-environment interaction. However, the consensus critique brings with it significant limitations, and consequently I contend that one important implication of this analysis is that the interests of population health would be well served by moving beyond the consensus critique.

Most critically, from a sociological perspective, the consensus critique offers a very partial and constrained analysis of the vulnerabilities of the environmental health sciences as a field. In claiming that further scientization—in this case, via the development of molecular techniques—can settle controversies about the effects of environmental exposures, the consensus critique diverts attention from the political and economic interests that motivate ongoing challenges to environmental health science. This is not to argue that it is possible or even desirable for the environmental health sciences to exist in some sort of purely autonomous state, removed from the contentious politics of environmental regulation. However, by translating political and economic issues into the logic and language of the scientific field, the consensus critique obfuscates the degree to which political and economic agendas are driving knowledge production in the environmental health sciences.

Related, promoting molecular technologies for their capacity to increase the certainty of environmental health research may have the unintended consequence of legitimizing industry's efforts to use uncertainty as a basis for questioning the validity of environmental epidemiology and toxicology. As historians of science Oreskes and Conway observe, doubt mongering relies on and propagates an erroneous view of science: "[I]f someone tells us that things are uncertain, we think that means that the science is muddled. This is a mistake" (2010: 34). However, uncertainty is part of scientific knowledge production; it does not indicate that the science is flawed (Michaels 2008: 165–166). Recognizing this, regulatory science has relied on a weight-of-evidence approach, as a way of "hedging" against the uncertainties inherent to any single epidemiological or toxicological study (Oreskes & Conway 2010: 142). By promising a molecular fix to problems of uncertainty, the consensus critique may have the unintended consequence of raising false expectations about scientific knowledge production and thereby further institutionalizing the vulnerability of the environmental health sciences.

It is time for an open dialogue among scientists, risk assessors, regulators, community groups, activists, and regulated industries about what certainty is or could be in the context of environmental health controversies. As suggested by scientists whom I interviewed, this conversation should include explicit consideration of differences in what certainty means across institutional domains within the environmental health arena:

> The basic scientist who deals with certainty—something has to be close to 100%. The toxicologists say, "Well that's not true, maybe 90% is good for me." And the policymaker might say, "Well, maybe 80% is good for me, because I have to make a decision. I have to make a decision on what's safe, I can't wait until all the information is in, so I want to use your system now to give me 80% confidence of what my decision is — for [a] safe exposure level (Interview S81).

A more open discourse about uncertainty in environmental health science should provide opportunities for communities, activists, and other stakeholders to articulate what level(s) of uncertainty are acceptable to them. In this way, abandoning the consensus critique might also open up new pathways for democratic participation in science.

At the same time, the narrow focus of the consensus critique excludes a broader set of questions about how human bodies come to be located in and affected by the environments in which they are embedded. To begin, the consensus critique, with its focus on the process of risk assessment, ignores entirely the social, political, and economic factors that make some people more likely to be exposed to environmental toxins. The agenda set by the consensus critique is unlikely therefore to do anything to address health disparities or issues of environmental injustice. Second, and related, the consensus critique is less concerned with what knowledge is needed to protect and improve public health than it is with what techniques will make toxicological risk assessment quicker, less expensive, and more robust to uncertainty campaigns and legal challenges. To be sure, public health would be well served by quick, affordable, and reliable assessments of environmental chemicals, especially given the thousands of chemicals for which toxicological data are not available. However, insofar as environmental health research is oriented to the regulatory paradigm—with its focus on isolating the effects of a single chemical exposure—it also is limited in its ability to speak to the effects of the complex environments in which our bodies are embedded. As such, moving beyond the consensus critique should open up space for questioning the assumption that experimental bioassay techniques offer the best means of assessing how complex environmental exposures actually affect the health of individuals and populations.

Moving beyond the consensus critique also will require an open debate in the environmental health sciences about whether, or to what extent, the information that will strengthen the empirical basis for environmental health risk assessment and regulation requires research on the cutting edge of molecular science. As one scientist asked pointedly, when it is clear that an exposure is harmful to human health, "Do you need to understand mechanisms to argue [that we need to] to reduce exposures?" (Interview S50). Likewise, as made vivid by the history of lead exposure among children in the United States, dramatic improvements in population health can be achieved when public policy is put in place to protect the entire population.

By offering a critique of this narrow consensus and by highlighting the importance of new foci for debate and contention in the environmental health arena, my hope is that this analysis will broaden ongoing debates about the future of environmental health research. Looking deep inside the human body and at events occurring at the molecular level provides fascinating insights into the pathways through which environmental exposures damage human bodies. Further, these molecular approaches promise to bolster, at least for a short while, the scientific authority of environmental health scientists, many of whom are deeply committed to public health. However, molecularization cannot remediate the structural vulnerabilities of the field of the environmental health sciences; these inhere not simply in its methods, but in its ties and exposure to other fields in the contentious politics of the environmental health arena. Nor can molecularization protect children like Sunday Abek, who are made vulnerable to poisons in their homes and communities by social, political, and economic conditions. The challenge—not just for environmental health scientists, but for all of us who care about population health—is to find new ways to address the structural vulnerabilities of the environmental health sciences, without ever losing sight of the lives and life chances of our most vulnerable citizens.

Afterword

HOW MUCH SCIENCE DOES A SOCIAL SCIENTIST
NEED TO KNOW?

I've been privileged to present my research to a wide variety of audiences over the past ten years. I've given talks to sociologists, environmental health scientists (at the NIEHS and elsewhere), historians of medicine, researchers who study the ethical, legal, and social implications of genetics, interdisciplinary groups focused on issues of science and justice, and population health researchers. As you would imagine, I get very different questions from these various audiences for my work, and this has been tremendously helpful to me in developing my analysis. In this afterword, I want to take up a line of inquiry that has arisen in almost all of these settings: what do sociologists who study science need to know about the science that they are studying?

The question of how much science one needs to know in order to do science and technology studies (STS) gets expressed in different ways, and these differences are telling. Sometimes I am asked how I figured out "how much" science I could learn without losing my critical perspective as a social scientist. This question assumes that understanding science from the perspective of scientists poses a threat to one's ability to do analysis; the implication is that doing science and technology studies requires that one be vigilant about not "going native" by taking on the worldview of one's subjects. Sometimes I am asked questions from a somewhat opposite point of view: Do I have a science background? And, if not, how did I develop sufficient technical expertise to understand the science that I study? These questions may derive from an assumption that sociological analysis of science requires that one be trained in the sciences; the implication is that doing science and technology studies requires that one "think like a scientist" about scientific research. Alternatively, they may merely point to a belief that social scientists need enough technical training to understand the workings of the science they are studying.

My approach takes a middle path between the two perspectives indexed by these questions. Because my research endeavors to understand transformations in environmental health science from the perspective of environmental health scientists (and policy makers, and activists), it was important to me to understand—to the best of my ability—the worldview of the people whom I was interviewing. As I began my dissertation research, I immersed myself in the relevant scientific literature. Later, I prepared for interviews by reading the publications of the scientists who had agreed to talk with me. As I conducted interviews—and throughout my postdoctoral training—I also attended ground rounds, scientific conferences and symposia, and audited classes in genetics and epidemiology. Further, during the summer of 2002, when I worked as an intern in the NIEHS Program in Environmental Health Policy and Ethics, I not only attended seminars designed to introduce interns to the work of the Institute, but also was privileged to be assigned a science mentor, who kindly took time out of his schedule each week to meet with me; between meetings, I read articles and observed laboratories to which he directed me. I took field notes in all of these settings, often focusing especially on ideas, objects, or goals that scientists seemed to take for granted that were new or strange to me. By making the concepts, objects, and assumptions of scientists' worldview explicit foci of my study, I was able to maintain critical distance, while building my understanding of environmental health science *from the perspective of environmental health scientists.* Indeed, I would encourage scholars of science and technology to use the process of learning science as a means of analysis. This requires extensive writing of field notes and analytic memos, so that one can trace changes in one's understanding of key concepts in the field under study, as well as the epistemologies undergirding them.

I previously had earned a masters in public health (MPH), which required that I take graduate-level courses in biostatistics, epidemiology, and environmental health science. This was a major contribution to my engagement with the scientists whom I study. Indeed, I often think of my MPH coursework as intensive language training, because it provided me with the basic vocabulary necessary to read journal articles and talk with environmental epidemiologists and toxicologists about their work. Although this level of technical background is not required by most STS research projects, my sense is that, alongside these purely functional advantages, having some shared language made scientists more comfortable talking with me.

To be sure, there is no *one* language of science. Anyone who has taken classes in biology and physics knows this to be true. However, even within the life sciences, languages vary. Indeed, as the scientists whom I interviewed made clear, molecularization in the environmental health sciences has required that toxicologists learn the language of genomics, and computational biologists learn the language of toxicology. My goal was to learn enough of each of these languages to talk with scientists with diverse disciplinary training and research practices. At the same time, struggling myself to learn these varied languages gave me an important perspective on the challenges that scientists face as well.

That said, taking the role of a novice in these interviews had real advantages. Even when I did have relevant background knowledge, I often put it aside, asking scientists to begin at the beginning and explain their research to me as if I was a student in an introductory-level class or a summer intern newly assigned to their lab. Such questions invited scientists to socialize me into their worldview as if I were one of their students. Although I do not think that these conversations could take the place of the extensive socialization that occurs during graduate training—which would include hands-on research experience, presenting at conferences, publishing in journals, and participating in journal clubs—they did help to sensitize me to the underlying logic of different fields of research. I must point out that I was consistently impressed by—and grateful for—environmental health scientists' ability to explain complex ideas and techniques in accessible ways.

I would argue that the fact that we ask these sorts of questions of sociologists who study science highlights two important issues for science and technology studies. First, it points to an underlying cultural assumption—among social scientists and life scientists alike—that science is a world or a culture apart from our daily lives. In fact, most social settings are far enough from our personal experience and knowledge that we must learn a good deal about them before entering their field to study them. However, very few sociologists who study English-speaking industrialized societies are asked to provide an account of how they learned what they needed to know to do their fieldwork (or, indeed, to provide a glossary of key terms for their readers). Relatedly, I have never been asked how I learned enough about issues of public policy or social justice to do interviews with policy makers or environmental justice activists. Of course, scientific terminology does, in fact, pervade our daily lives; one can hardly listen to the evening news without hearing both literal and metaphoric uses of scientific concepts. However, part of the authority of the scientific field derives from its specialized knowledge, which functions as a barrier to entry. As such, credible claims to having gained meaningful access to the field require assurances that one is in possession of a more advanced proficiency (even if not sufficiently advanced to have the capital to successfully make claims in the field itself). Second, and more practically, these questions point to some of the real challenges facing scholars of science, technology, and medicine. I still remember vividly a seminar at UCSF, in which Professor Emeritus Elliott Friedson explained to us that one of the reasons he had stopped doing research on the medical profession per se (after his hugely important and influential study, *Profession of Medicine*) was that he was no longer willing to keep up with the relevant literature in both medicine *and* sociology. Similarly, the sciences that I study are constantly changing, and keeping up with advances in scientific field—while maintaining my primary focus in sociology—has required significant amounts of time and energy. That said, for those of us who are deeply committed to carving out space for new forms of public discourse about science, health, and social justice, these challenges are well worth undertaking.

APPENDIX A: Data and Methods

This analysis draws on data from a multisited ethnographic project conducted in two stages from September 2000 through July 2004.[1] In contrast to a more traditional ethnographic approach, multisite ethnography "moves out from the single sites and local situations of conventional ethnographic research designs to examine the circulation of cultural meanings, objects, and identities in diffuse time [and] space" (Marcus 1995/1998: 79). It is a methodology well suited to following complex cultural objects, such as scientific concepts or technologies, across multiple locations and constituencies (Rapp 1999: 3). Across locations, I both conducted interviews, and, whenever possible, participant observation. To clarify the nature of my primary data (Duneier 1999), I distinguish "interviews" from "field notes" in parentheses following quotations in the text. While I conducted a few interviews with scientists based in Canada and Europe, all of my fieldwork was conducted in the United States.

The first set of data upon which I draw is in-depth qualitative interviews ($n = 81$). The majority of my interviews were with scientists formally educated in molecular biology, genetics, epidemiology, toxicology, pharmacology, and preventive medicine who now work in the environmental health sciences, including the emerging subfields of molecular epidemiology, environmental genomics, and toxicogenomics ($n = 50$). In addition, I interviewed regulatory scientists and administrators based at the U.S. Environmental Protection Agency and the Food and Drug Administration ($n = 7$). Finally, I was able to interview several scientists working in the pharmaceutical and biotech industries ($n = 5$). Most interviews were 60–90 minutes in duration, with some as long as 120 minutes. With few exceptions, the interviews with scientists were recorded and transcribed verbatim.

Environmental health scientists, regulators, and administrators were initially identified via a comprehensive literature review and from the participant lists of environmental health conferences and symposia (see below), which allowed me to map the arena of concern (Clarke 2005: 137–138). Purposive sampling was used as themes began to emerge from my coding of interview data (Charmaz 2006); for example, as it became clear that there was very little open dissent regarding research on gene-environment interaction, I began to ask respondents to suggest which of their colleagues were more critical of the molecular turn in the environmental health sciences.

I conducted a second set of interviews with environmental health and justice activists and community organizers ($n = 6$). These interviews tended to be less formal than the interviews with scientists. Often, they blurred the lines between "interview" and "participant observation" because many took place during community events or over lunch. Additionally, almost all of these respondents requested that I not audiotape our conversation. Because of the reluctance of activists to be interviewed "on the record," I relied more heavily on participant observation in gathering data on activists' perspectives and concerns.

I've assigned numbers to each interview, to protect the confidentiality of my respondents. In addition to a number, interviews with scientists working in universities, the NIH, and the pharmaceutical industry are labeled with an S. Interviews with regulatory scientists and administrators working in the regulatory agencies and with activists are labeled with a P. I recognize that this rather simplistic labeling might obscure differences in the positions of those whose words I am quoting. However, the fact that many of the scientists I interviewed in pharma were once employed in government or academic research institutions, and a few of the regulators were formerly activists, raises concerns both about classification and "internal confidentiality" that cannot be otherwise addressed (Tolich 2004).[2]

The second major source of data utilized in this analysis comes from ethnographic observation. From 2000 to 2004, I conducted observation at meetings sponsored by the National Institutes of Health, Environmental Protection Agency, Society of Toxicology, American Association of Cancer Research, and West Harlem Environmental Action. At these meetings, I took notes both on formal presentations and on lunchtime conversations and corridor talk. I also spent time "hanging out" with scientists whom I had formally interviewed at other times. In fact, I was quite grateful for their willingness to talk with me in these less formal settings and introduce me to their colleagues. The introduction often began, "This is the person I was telling you about, who insisted that I sign an informed consent form!" As noted, I also attended community health fairs and protests, at the invitation of environmental health and justice activists in the San Francisco Bay Area and in New York City. In all cases, I was completely forthcoming in my interactions about my purpose in being at the meeting, fair, or protest.

I conducted participant observation also at the National Institute of Environmental Health Sciences (NIEHS). First, in 2002, I worked full-time at the NIEHS as a summer intern in the Program on Environmental Health Policy and Ethics. My primary responsibility as an intern was to serve as a liaison to the Ethical, Legal, and Social Implications (ELSI) Working Group of the National Center for Toxicogenomics, which gave me a remarkable vantage point on the efforts of NIEHS scientists and their allies to establish toxicogenomics as a new basis for environmental risk assessment and regulation. In 2003–2004, I returned to the NIEHS, for one week of every month, as a postdoctoral fellow in the Office of

NIH History, which provided me with the opportunity to conduct new interviews (n = 13) and participant observation. During this time, I also reinterviewed a subset of my original respondents (n = 10); these interviews allowed me the opportunity to bring my analysis back to my informants and to gain further insights, both as they responded to my analysis and updated me on recent events and initiatives.

Finally, this analysis draws on journal articles, conference proceedings, policy reports, congressional statements, and other archival materials. Articles from the peer-reviewed literature in the environmental health sciences were identified during two different reviews, one in 2000 and another in 2008, using key words such as "gene-environment interaction," "environmental genomics, "molecular epidemiology," and "toxicogenomics." The library of the NIEHS proved a rich site for locating archival materials about the Institute's founding, development, and current initiatives. Conference proceedings and policy reports were identified during both participant observation and in interviews, with many respondents generously providing me with copies of these documents.

All of the data were analyzed using modified grounded theory and analytical-induction approach (Timmermans & Tavory 2007). First, the empirical material was systematically coded in dialogue with a close reading of salient themes in the literature of both sociology and science and technology studies (STS). Second, I treated environmental genomics (Chapter 3), molecular epidemiology (Chapter 4), and toxicogenomics (Chapter 5) as "cases" that could be compared to each other, providing additional analytic leverage and explanatory power (Glaser & Strauss 1967; Ragin 1992).

Notes

INTRODUCTION

1.   The paint on the porch was 37% lead by weight. House paint contained up to 50% lead before 1955. Federal law lowered the amount of lead allowable in paint to 1% in 1971 and to 0.06% (600 ppm by dry weight) in 1977.
   At URL: http://www.atsdr.cdc.gov/csem/csem.asp?csem=7&po=8. See also: http://grist.org/article/spin2/ (accessed July 2010).

2.   The National Academy of Sciences warns that levels as low as 10 micrograms of lead per deciliter ($\mu g/dL$) of blood in infants, children, and pregnant women are associated with impairments in cognitive function, fetal organ development, intelligence, hearing, as well as behavior difficulties (NAS 1993). Based on an international study of children who were followed from infancy until they were five to ten years of age, environmental health scientists have concluded that there is no safe level of lead exposure for children (Lanphear, et al. 2005). In May 2012, in response to what its Advisory Committee on Childhood Lead Poisoning Prevention called "compelling evidence that BLLs lower than 10 $\mu g/dL$ are associated with IQ deficits, attention-related behaviors, and poor academic

achievement," the Centers for Disease Control and Prevention (CDC) abandoned the 10 µg threshold of concern in favor of a new level based on the U.S. population of children ages one to five years who are in the top 2.5% of children when tested for lead in their blood (when compared to children who are exposed to more lead than most children). At URL: http://www.cdc.gov/nceh/lead/ACCLPP/Lead_Levels_in_Children_Fact_Sheet.pdf (accessed June 27, 2012).

3. At URL: http://www.atsdr.cdc.gov/toxprofiles/tp13.pdf (accessed June 27, 2012). On the greater susceptibility of children to lead poisoning, see especially pp. 220–224, 363–374.

4. Secondary prevention—programs that seek to identify and treat children who have been exposed to lead, before it causes irreparable damage—are also an important part of efforts to prevent lead poisoning. In 1988, the Lead Contamination Control Act authorized the CDC to initiate and coordinate efforts to eliminate childhood lead poisoning in the United States. The CDC provides funding to state and local health departments to determine the extent of childhood lead poisoning by screening children for elevated blood lead levels, helping to ensure that lead-poisoned infants and children receive medical and environmental follow-up, developing neighborhood-based efforts to prevent childhood lead poisoning, and educating the public and health-care providers about childhood lead poisoning.

5. It took more than twenty years for this phaseout to be complete; as of 1995, lead was no longer allowed in gasoline.

6. In 2003, the CDC estimated that approximately 250,000 U.S. children aged one to five years have blood lead levels greater than 10 µg/dL (CDC 2003).

7. See also URL: http://www.cdc.gov/mmwr/preview/mmwrhtml/mm5402a4.htm.

8. The President's Task Force on Environmental Health Risks and Safety Risks to Children was established in April 1997 by Executive Order 13045. It was cochaired by the Secretary of the Department of Health and Human Services and the Administrator of the Environmental Protection Agency and included sixteen departments and White House offices. At URL: http://yosemite.epa.gov/ochp/ochpweb.nsf/content/whatwe_fedtask.htm. See President's Task Force on Environmental Health Risks and Safety Risks to Children. 2000. *Eliminating Childhood Lead Poisoning: A Federal Strategy Targeting Lead Paint Hazards.* At URL: http://yosemite.epa.gov/ochp/ochpweb.nsf/content/leadhaz.htm/$file/leadhaz.pdf (accessed July 21, 2010).

9. As a consequence of the success of efforts to reduce lead exposure in the United States, researchers who study lead often conduct research in other countries (Interviews S04, S06, S11).

10. For definitions of medical and scientific terms throughout the book, please see the Glossary.

11. Markowitz and Rosner (2002) provide a detailed historical account of this strategy. Proctor (1995), Brandt (2007), and Oreskes and Conway (2010)

detail how the tobacco industry promoted the idea that genetic susceptibility—rather than smoking—is the real cause of lung cancer.

12.   A detailed description of my research methods can be found in Appendix A.

13.   I was not successful in my attempts to interview scientists working in chemical industry–sponsored research, although I conducted several interviews with scientists working in the pharmaceutical and biotech industries. This analysis therefore relies heavily on archival analyses of industry's efforts to generate controversy and create uncertainty about the health and environmental effects of specific products. I draw especially on recent books by historians Brandt (2007), Markowitz and Rosner (2002), Oreskes and Conway (2010), and Proctor (1995).

14.   Auyero and Swistun (2009) provide an especially compelling, and devastating, analysis of the ways that uncertainty shapes the possibilities of individual and collective action in the context of toxic pollution.

15.   Rushefsky (1986) was one of the first to observe that stakeholders use uncertainty as a resource in their efforts to influence policy.

16.   Over 90% of American respondents report genetic makeup as at least somewhat important for physical illness, and almost two-thirds do for success in life (Shostak et al. 2009).

17.   I borrow this metaphor from Bearman (2005).

18.   I appreciate that these ways of "doing" social science are not often, or perhaps easily, combined. However, along with my colleagues in science, technology, and medicine studies, I find that "bringing literatures together is a crucial task for scholars concerned with key features of the modern world" (Epstein 2007: 18).

19.   As argued by Levi Martin (2003) and Panofsky (2011), the analytic categories proffered by Bourdieu can be useful for empirical analysis, even if one rejects his relativist and normative stance.

20.   Bourdieu most often wrote about science as a homogeneous social field, in contradistinction to other fields of social production (1975). As Sismondo notes, "Although Bourdieu's fields often map roughly onto scientific fields, the former is not defined in disciplinary terms, but is rather a space of engagement or a structure of relationships that bounds the practices of someone interested in contributing . . ." (2011: 2). In contrast, congruent with recent work in the sociology of science (Hess 2011; Lave 2012; Panofsky 2011), my analysis uses this approach to examine specific scientific fields. As Camic notes, the autonomization of a field takes place through the creation of disciplines (2011: 278).

21.   Moore (2008) skillfully challenges the assumption that scientists' interest in establishing their expertise and authority will always trump other motivations. Moreover, as we will see, some commitments of environmental

health scientists—i.e., contributing to highly politicized regulatory processes—simultaneously affirm and undermine their expertise.

22. Sociologists offer varied definitions of "arenas." My use of this term build on Jasper's conceptualization of arenas as "sets of resources and rules that channel contention into certain kinds of actions and offer rewards and outcomes" (2004: 5) and symbolic interactionist understandings of arenas as existing when diverse stakeholders "that focus on a given issue and are prepared to act in some way together" (Strauss et al. 1964: 377; see also Clarke 1998).

23. Fligstein and McAdam offer three sets of binary distinctions to characterize the relationships between fields, which may be (1) distant or proximate, (2) vertical or horizontal, and (3) state or nonstate (2011: 8).

24. Panofsky (2011) and Sismondo (2011) eloquently articulate the importance of examining empirically the boundaries and autonomy of scientific fields. The foundational work on the boundaries of science, more broadly, is Gieryn (1999).

25. In fact, Bourdieu's fields analysis may be "completed, not contravened" in analyses that look at fields in terms of interinstitutional relations (John Levi Martin 2003: 26). Bourdieu theorizes scientific institutions as the objectification of the outcome of previous struggles and allows that scientific institutions may be protagonists in subsequent struggles (1975: 27). However, his writings about the scientific field emphasize the strategies of researchers, much more than they attend to the dynamics between institutions. As Sismondo puts it, "Bourdieu's sociology of science, while it aims to explain scientific knowledge, is a sociology of scientists" (2009: 11).

26. Understanding the arrangements of social actors in particular institutions is an important part of explaining "why, acting as they do, individuals bring about the social outcomes they do" (Hedstrom & Bearman 2009: 8; see also Abbott 1997).

27. According to Bourdieu, the overall autonomy of the field is defined by "the extent to which it manages to impose its own norms and sanctions on the whole set of producers" (Bourdieu 1983: 321). At the same time, the internal structure of the field also is structured by an axis defined by an autonomous and a heteronomous pole. At the autonomous end of any field are those actors whose production is controlled most thoroughly by the forms of capital specific to that field. At the heteronomous end are those whose production is shaped primarily by outside forces. In fields that are less autonomous, the tension between actors at the autonomous and heteronomous poles of the fields provide a motor for change (Bourdieu 1996: 121).

28. As John Levi Martin notes, often "the only way to reach conditions that we cognize and wish for is to make use of those conditions that we have not wished for" (Levi Martin 2003: 44).

29. I adapted these questions from Fligstein (2001), which was the only writing on "socially skilled actors" available to me while doing the research and

analysis; I have benefited, however, from reading his more recent work with McAdam on this topic (2011; 2012).

30. The association between environmental health science and public health—rather than clinical biomedicine—is an important example of how history matters in this story.

31. Fligstein & McAdam suggest that realist case studies of fields are often "a kind of sociological history" (2012: 184).

32. There is wide variation in how social scientists conceptualize path dependence (Pierson 2000: 252–253; Thelen 2003: 221). As a consequence of this variation, path dependence may appear as either pervasive in society and politics or as an extremely rare occurrence (Thelen 1999: 220).

33. At URL: http://www.nytimes.com/2009/05/14/us/14plastic.html?ref= bisphenol_a (accessed July 2, 2010).

34. At URL: http://www.nytimes.com/2010/06/16/us/16cell.html?fta=y (accessed July 2, 2010).

35. At URL: http://www.nytimes.com/2008/04/18/business/18plastic.html? ref=bisphenol_a (accessed July 2, 2010).

36. At URL: http://www.nytimes.com/2010/03/12/science/earth/12zero .html?fta=y (accessed July 2, 2010).

37. The National Toxicology Program (NTP) has ongoing research on both bisphenol-A and cell phones. See http://www.niehs.nih.gov/health/docs/bpa-factsheet.pdf and http://www.niehs.nih.gov/health/docs/cell-phone-fact-sheet .pdf (accessed July 2, 2010).

38. http://www.nytimes.com/2009/12/17/us/17water.html (accessed July 2, 2010).

39. http://www.nytimes.com/2008/01/23/dining/23sushi.html?ref=mercury_ in_tuna (accessed July 2, 2010).

40. http://www.nytimes.com/2005/07/07/fashion/thursdaystyles/07skin .html?scp=1&sq=%22cosmetic+safety+%22&st=nyt (accessed July 2, 2010).

41. Regulatory institutions, by contrast, have been studied more extensively (Carpenter 2010; Jasanoff 1990, 1995).

42. By *institutionalization*, I refer to the activities and mechanisms by which structures, models, rules, and problem-solving routines become established as a taken for granted part of everyday social reality (Campbell 2005).

43. At URL: http://www.genome.gov/19518663 (accessed October 31, 2012).

44. As possible, I will provide a short description of the background and/ or current position of the scientists whom I quote directly. However, for two reasons, these descriptions should be viewed as partial. First, if I were to provide a detailed and complete description of each scientist's educational background and training, I would compromise the confidentiality that I promised my interviewees. Second, although environmental epidemiology and toxicology are at

the center of the environmental health sciences, they attract researchers with backgrounds in other fields, including biochemistry, biostatistics, molecular biology, genetics, pathology, pharmacology, preventive medicine, and veterinary medicine. As such, many environmental health scientists have complex backgrounds and career trajectories that defy short descriptors; for example, what is the correct description of a scientist who holds a PhD in molecular biology, describes his research interests as "protein chemistry and cell biology," and is a tenured professor in a department of toxicology? Or, a scientist who holds a PhD in toxicology and works in a department of environmental health science but comments that "I have always been a molecular biologist"? When an interviewee specifically names his or her field, I use that description. I have also gathered information on scientists' educational backgrounds and training from their websites and curriculum vitae. However, even as I attend to these differences, I argue that their shared location in the environmental health arena powerfully affects the research practices of these scientists.

45.   See, for example: http://www.ph.ucla.edu/moltox/index.php (accessed July 9, 2010).

46.   Testimony of Dr. Samuel Wilson, Acting Director of the National Institute of Environmental Health Sciences, September 2007.

47.   See Chapter 5 for a detailed discussion of Tox21.

48.   In addition to genomics, the workshop considered associated technologies focused on mRNA (transcriptomics), proteins (proteomics), metabolites (metabonomics), and the effects of stressors on gene expressions (toxicogenomics).

49.   National Toxicology Program Toxicity Reports [abstracts and full reports] are available at http://ehp.niehs.nih.gov/ntp/docs/toxreports.html (accessed July 9, 2010).

CHAPTER ONE

1.   NAEHSC is a Congressionally mandated body that advises the secretary of Health and Human Services, the director of the National Institutes of Health, and the director of the NIEHS on matters relating to the direction of research, research support, training, and career development supported by the NIEHS. At URL: http://www.niehs.nih.gov/about/orgstructure/boards/naehsc/index .cfm (accessed May 14, 2010).

2.   Dr. David Schwartz was the Director of the NIEHS from May 2005 to August 2007. At the time of this hearing, he was under investigation for having violated the NIH's rules regarding conflict of interest. He did not return to the NIEHS.

3. The implied contrast here is with other National Institutes of Health, such as the National Cancer Institute or the National Heart, Lung, and Blood Institute, which are defined by their focus on particular diseases and organs.

4. Put differently, the environmental health sciences are shaped by outside forces and thus are relatively less autonomous (Bourdieu 1996).

5. At URL: http://www.niehs.nih.gov/about/od/strategicplan/stakeholder-community-workshop/index.cfm (accessed October 13, 2011).

6. On mapping arenas, see Clarke (2005).

7. At URL: http://www.niehs.nih.gov/home.htm (accessed July 2002). This mission is subject to minor revisions. In 2009, the NIEHS webpage stated, "The mission of the NIEHS is to reduce the burden of human illness and disability by understanding how the environment influences the development and progression of human disease." At URL: http://www.niehs.nih.gov/ (accessed July 2009).

8. In comparison, the budget for the National Cancer Institute in 2005 was $4.9 billion. At URL: http://www.cancer.gov/aboutnci/directorscorner/jen/cancerresearch-2-1-07. NIEHS budget information for 2005 is available at URL: http://www.hhs.gov/budget/testify/b20040401q.html (accessed May 25, 2010).

9. The EJ and CBPR programs of the NIEHS are described later in this chapter and in Chapter 6. EHP is located online at URL: http://ehp03.niehs.nih.gov/home.action (accessed November 23, 2011).

10. Even as environmental health scientists have taken up broader definitions of the environment and included behavioral and lifestyle factors in their research, how to study and engage with broader social and political definitions of the environment clearly poses challenges. As a NIEHS administrator commented, "our [NIH's] culture and historical method of doing research has been to understand basic mechanisms and to make use of that information in translational approaches that benefit public health" (Interview S87).

11. Conversely, a cancer researcher complained in an interview that the NIEHS's focus on gene-environment interaction reflected its jurisdictional ambitions rather than the state of science about human cancer causation: "Their whole mantra is the environment because that's what they get funded to study and they prefer a very vague, loose definition of the term, because then anything is . . . a candidate. But that's not what we know about human cancer causation; it's not so vague and imprecise. So that's why I don't like the term, because it's not a scientific term in the sense that it means anything relative to human cancer" (Interview S18).

12. At URL: http://www.gei.nih.gov/exposurebiology/index.asp (accessed June 13, 2007).

13. At URL: http://www.gei.nih.gov/exposurebiology/funding.asp (accessed June 13, 2007).

14. These tensions in the environmental health sciences echo—and recapitulate—debates in the social sciences about the "structure of poverty" and

the "culture of poverty" as causes of ongoing poverty and poor health in inner-city neighborhoods. See, for example, http://www.nytimes.com/2010/10/18/us/18poverty.html. I thank David Pellow for challenging me to think about the extent to which molecularized views of bodies, environments, and their interactions articulate with resurgent interest in cultural explanations of health disparities.

15. The mandate for the Report on Carcinogens is in Section 301(b)(4) of the Public Health Services Act of 1978. In 1993, Public Law 95-622 was amended to change the frequency of publication from an annual to a biennial report. At URL: http://ntp.niehs.nih.gov/?objectid=72016291-BDB7-CEBA-FEE1EA2A-11509B3A (accessed May 25, 2010).

16. At URL: http://www.niehs.nih.gov/about/od/director/index.cfm (accessed June 2009).

17. Additionally, as demonstrated in Chapter 5, environmental health scientists, in both government and academia, may join together to convince the regulatory agencies that they need particular kinds of information—for example, data on gene-environment interaction—in order to meet their mandates.

18. This mandate applied also to the older FDA and the Occupational Health and Safety Administration (OSHA), the agencies responsible for the regulation and safety of drugs, biological products, medical devices, our nation's food supply, cosmetics, products that emit radiation, and our nation's workplaces.

19. At URL: http://www.epa.gov/hg/regs.htm#laws (accessed June 2009).

20. At URL: http://www.epa.gov/osw/hazard/tsd/mercury/laws.htm (accessed June 2009).

21. At URL: http://www.fda.gov/oc/opacom/mehgadvisory1208.html (accessed October 16, 2007). For a comprehensive history of the FDA, see Carpenter (2010).

22. At URL: http://www.cpsc.gov/cpscpub/pubs/5057.html (accessed April 2010).

23. At URL: http://www.epa.gov/OSA/pdfs/ratf-final.pdf (accessed May 2008).

24. Such cases often involve emergency circumstances. For example, individuals who live near nuclear power plants may be provided with potassium iodine tablets. Potassium iodine inhibits radioiodine uptake by the thyroid gland, under certain specified conditions of use, and may thereby reduce the risk of thyroid cancer in the event of accidental radiation exposure.

25. Traditional measures of productivity, such as number of publications and impact factors, are also tracked by the NIEHS. Dr. Ben Van Houten, in the NIEHS Division of Extramural Research, developed an assessment model for grant-funded research that has since been adopted throughout the NIH. At URL: http://nihrecord.od.nih.gov/newsletters/03_05_2002/story04.htm (accessed July 2002).

26.   For detailed case studies of this strategy, see Brandt (2007), Markowitz and Rosner (2002), Michaels (2008), Ong and Glantz (2001), Oreskes and Conway (2010), and Proctor (1995).

27.   See, as examples, the Chemical Industry Institute of Toxicology at URL: http://www.thehamner.org/institutes/ciit/ (accessed June 2009) and the Silent Spring Institute at URL: http://www.silentspring.org/ (accessed June 2009).

28.   All data cited in this section from the ACC's website. At URL: http://www.americanchemistry.com/ (accessed July 3, 2012).

29.   At URL: http://www.niehs.nih.gov/research/supported/programs/justice/index.cfm (accessed July 2009).

30.   Ibid.

31.   The case studies in this collection simultaneously highlight the profound cultural and institutional challenges to such transformation.

32.   I do not mean to suggest that all stakeholders are equally able to pose serious challenges to environmental health science. To be sure, the financial and scientific resources available to the chemical industry dwarf those of the EJM. Likewise, the staffing, priorities, and possibilities afforded to regulatory agencies under different administrations may shape their receptivity to certain kinds of challenges. Some of the first case studies on this topic appear in Jasanoff (1990, 1995). Ottinger and Cohen (2010) provide more recent case studies focused explicitly on EJ activists. However, research is needed to systematically characterize successful challenges to scientific expertise in the environmental health arena.

33.   This push to focus on mechanisms reflected trends in toxicology at the time, as a famously iconoclastic (and controversial) toxicologist noted: "toxicologists today worship at the altar of mechanism, and that is all they talk about, just mechanism, mechanism, mechanism. The only thing that counts is mechanism, mechanism, mechanism" (Interview 03).

34.   This hierarchy has extended also within NIEHS and NTP, with a "historical division . . . between the NTP and everyone else. There used to be a separate NTP division that consisted of all the chemistry, pathology, and toxicology involved in testing, in programmatic research. And then the DIR [Division of Intramural Research] had the 'real scientists' who did real research, basic research that was investigator initiated, rather than programmatic" (Field Notes, NIEHS 2002). Dr. Olden reorganized the two institutions in the early years of his tenure as director and brought the NTP scientists into the DIR (Stone 1993). However, at the NIEHS "there is still a sense of esoteric, basic versus applied, mission-based research" (Field Notes, NIEHS 2002). Shapin (2008) provides a compelling history of these categories in the life sciences more broadly.

35.   Of course, there are alternative explanations for the perceived marginalization of environmental health sciences in the mid-1990s. For example, in

1994, the Republican-controlled Congress explicitly targeted both environmental health research and regulation for reductions in funding. It was quite striking that *none* of the scientists I interviewed referred to the political climate of the mid-1990s in their accounts of the development of their research agendas. In contrast, environmental regulators pointed directly to the pressures being felt by their agencies as Republicans began to implement their Contract with America.

36.   At URL: http://www.cdc.gov/genomics/about/reports/1997.htm (accessed July 19, 2010).

37.   Abstracts for the papers presented at these conferences are available online at URL: http://www.cdc.gov/genomics/about/achievements.htm (accessed July 19, 2010).

38.   At URL: http://www.cdc.gov/genomics/about/reports/1997.htm (accessed July 19, 2010).

39.   It also fits well with neoliberal approaches to public health (Peterson & Lupton 1996).

40.   In fields analysis, as in neoinstitutional theory, the transformation of fields is seen as more likely when current arrangements start to break down, whether due to events that destabilize existing institutions and/or endogenous processes stemming from some serious crisis in the functioning of the current field (Fligstein 2001:109).

CHAPTER TWO

1.   Sociologists have made similar arguments (Pescosolido 2006).

2.   Drawing on the literature on social movements, as well as an inductive analysis of myriad cases of the transformation of scientific and intellectual fields, Frickel and Gross propose that the success of scientists' and intellectuals' movements (SIMs) hinges on actors having a complaint regarding the central intellectual tendencies of their field, access to key resources (e.g., employment, intellectual prestige, mobilizing structures), access to places where participants can be recruited, and a means of inspiring participants to embrace the claims of the SIM, such that they are willing to engage in collective action 2005).

3.   I borrow the concept of collective action frames from the literature on social movements, as well as more recent writings on scientists' social movements (Benford & Snow 2000; Benford 1993). Interestingly, scientists also refer to "framing" in their writings about the future of toxicology testing (Krewski et al. 2009: 475).

4.   In contrast, social movement frames often identify injustices, denote a sense of collective efficacy, and define the "others" against which collective action must be mobilized (Polletta 1998: 139).

5.   Many of these specific critiques have been used previously to mobilize environmental health scientists around emergent technologies. Genetically modified mouse models are another fairly recent example (Shostak 2007).

6.   Oreskes and Conway (2010) provide extensive historical evidence for this claim.

7.   In Chapter 5, we will see this approach at the center of the regulatory agencies' efforts to transform risk assessment (e.g., Krewski et al. 2009).

8.   In the following chapters, I describe the deep epistemological roots of each definition of gene-environment interaction.

9.   During several interviews, environmental health scientists drew this figure for me as a means explaining why they are interested in genetic variation in susceptibility to exposures. It appears also in the published literature (Puga et al. 1996).

10.   Research on environmental mutagenesis originally focused on the threat of environmental chemicals to future generations (i.e., via germ cell mutations); however, the effects of environmental exposures on somatic cells was a loosely related concern (Frickel 2004).

11.   The theory that mutagenesis was associated with carcinogenesis had existed since the 1920s. That chemicals could cause mutations was established in the work of Charlotte Auerbach and John M. Robson in the 1940s; by the 1960s, scientists had observed that some chemical carcinogens interact with DNA. For an incisive history of research on mutagenesis, see Frickel (2004).

12.   Such efforts are described in detail in Chapter 5.

13.   This is not to say that environmental health scientists are indifferent to issues of environmental justice. In fact, at the federal level, the NIEHS has been a leader in supporting research on environmental injustice, including partnerships with affected communities (Interview 37; Field Notes June 2002; Brown 2007).

14.   "Certain disadvantaged ethnic groups may have a higher incidence of certain susceptibility genes that render them more vulnerable to adverse effects of the environments they inhabit" write Olden and White (2005). As shown in Chapter 6, such statements represent the worst fears of EJ activists.

CHAPTER THREE

1.   For an important analysis of how timing of exposure became a central concern of environmental health science, see Vogel (2008).

2. For a comprehensive discussion of this strategy in other domains of biomedicine, see Lindee (2005).

3. These conceptualizations of bodily constitutions varied both by national context and by discipline (Mendelsohn 2001).

4. As I describe in detail in the following chapter, in contrast to their physician colleagues, nineteenth century public health reformers argued precisely that environmental factors were an independent and primary cause of illness in the population. In contrast, eugenic scientists argued that environmental and behavior "masked" the inherited, constitutional causes of disease (e.g., Brandt 2007: 176).

5. At the time that Garrod began his work, the terms *gene* and *genetics* did not exist (Motulsky 2002). However, Garrod corresponded with William Bateson, who noted that the patterning of such traits in families was consistent with the principles of Mendelian recessive inheritance (Harper 2005; Motulsky 2002). Scientists now refer to Garrod's work on alcaptonuria as the first proof of Mendelian genetics in humans (Mancinelli, Cronin, & Sadee 2000).

6. Clinical ecologists also have invoked the concept of biochemical individuality in their efforts to legitimize their approaches for assessing and treating people who experience the constellation of symptoms known as multiple chemical sensitivity (MCS) (Murphy 2006: 163).

7. Individual case reporting preceded this research. The first report of the potential danger of hemolytic anemia as a response to the antimalarial drug pamaquine was published in a case report in 1926, and reports of many similar individual cases followed (see Tarlov et al. 1962).

8. Such experimental strategies were not uncommon prior to the establishment of Institutional Review Boards and standardized federal ethics guidelines, under which prisoners are recognized as a vulnerable population deserving of protection against exploitation in human subjects research.

9. Scientists now recognize that G6PD deficiency, the cause of this susceptibility, is widely distributed among populations historically exposed to falciprum malaria. Like the trait for sickle cell anemia, the G6PD trait appears to confer some protection against malaria and is more common among people descended from areas where malaria is endemic (Calabrese 1996).

10. This focus has shifted in recent years, as pharmacogenetic and pharmacogenomic research increasingly is oriented toward the development of drugs for populations carrying specific genetic traits and/or developing tests for such traits (i.e., to identify drug targets or to improve the safety and efficacy of extant drugs) (Hedgecoe 2004).

11. The application of ecogenetics in industrial settings became a contentious political issue in 1980, when a four-part story in the *New York Times* problematized the lack of any consistent policy toward genetic testing in the

workplace, the apparent inconsistencies in screening practices across industries, and the lacunae in the scientific evidence base that proponents were using to advocate for such screening (Calabrese 1986: 1098; Nelkin 1989: 97). In the late 1990s, court cases against companies' use of genetic testing (often without the knowledge or informed consent of workers) brought renewed attention to workplace testing for genetic susceptibility. In 2008, the Genetic Information Nondiscrimination Act (GINA), which had been debated in Congress for 13 years, was signed into law; it prohibits health insurers and employers from discriminating on the basis of genetic information. At URL: http://frwebgate.access.gpo.gov/cgi-bin/getdoc.cgi?dbname=110_cong_bills&docid=f:h493enr.txt.pdf (accessed May 2010).

12. The National Advisory Environmental Health Sciences Council granted clearance for the Environmental Genome Project in February of 1998.

13. Environmental Genome Project website (accessed September 1999).

14. The term *genome* was coined by H. Winkler in 1920 to signify the complete set of human chromosomes and their genes. *Genomics* refers to the discipline that studies chromosomes and their genes (Olden & Guthrie 2001: 6).

15. The achievement of new work objects is often accomplished through their articulation with and through extant standards, objects, and practices (Fujimura 1996; Timmermans & Berg 1997). Moreover, new units of analysis are often developed in and from previous experimental systems (Fujimura 1996: 3).

16. Scientists were surprised to discover that the human genome contains far fewer genes than they had predicted. Environmental health scientists have used this fact to highlight the importance of gene-environment interaction for understanding human health and illness (Olden & White 2005).

17. All the SNP data generated by the Environmental Genome Project is stored on the GeneSNPs website. It is also deposited in the Genbank/NCBI dbSNPs database.

18. In the late 1980s, a convergence of advances in developmental, reproductive, and molecular biology made it possible for scientists to mutate or cause a loss of function in specific genes (Gordon 1989). Using targeted mutations in transgenic mice, scientists began to develop knockout mouse models of human disease to test the role of specific genes in disease etiology and progression (Smithies & Kim 1994).

19. As described in Chapter 6, the possibility that environmental genomics will shift the locus of responsibility for environmental health and illness to the individual level is a primary concern of environmental health and justice activists.

20. In 2006, Health and Human Services Secretary Mike Leavitt announced that the president's budget proposal for fiscal year (FY) 2007 would include $68 million for the Genes and Environment Initiative (GEI), a collaborative

project to combine genetic analysis and environmental technology development to understand how gene-environment interactions contribute to the etiology of common diseases.

21. At URL: http://www.niehs.nih.gov/research/supported/programs/egp/ (accessed October 8, 2009).

22. Given the subsequent advent of genome-wide association studies (GWAS), these numbers may appear small; recall, however, that the project was based rather on a candidate gene approach.

23. In collaboration with the National Human Genome Research Institute, the National Center for Biotechnology Information established the db-SNP database to serve as a central, public repository SNP data from around the world. At URL: http://www.ncbi.nlm.nih.gov/projects/SNP/get_html.cgi?whichHtml=overview, (accessed 10/8/2009).

24. Francis S. Collins was the Director of the NHGRI from 1993 to 2008. In 2009, President Barack Obama nominated Collins as Director of the NIH, a post to which he was confirmed soon thereafter.

25. At URL: http://www.niehs.nih.gov/about/od/programs/index.cfm#exposure (accessed October 8, 2009).

CHAPTER FOUR

1. Quoted in Revkin (2001).

2. This chapter draws extensively on three excellent histories of environmental health research (Murphy 2006; Nash 2006; Sellers 1997).

3. My analytic focus on visibility is informed especially by the work of Murphy (2006) on *regimes of perceptibility*.

4. Theories of the environmental causation of disease date to Hippocrates who, in the fifth century BCE, opined that "whoever wishes to investigate medicine properly" must attend to specific location in which people are living, including the temperature, winds, relation to the rising and setting sun, and the source and quality of water. Hippocrates focused also on human behaviors, including "whether they are fond of drinking and eating to excess, and given to indolence, or are fond of exercise and labor, and not given to excess in eating and drinking" (Section 1, translated by F. Adams). At URL: http://classics.mit.edu/Hippocrates/airwatpl.1.1.html (accessed February 17, 2010)

5. Filth was also seen by some Sanitarians, including William Farr, as a basis for active pathogenic "ferments" (Paneth et al. 1998: 1545; see also Parodi, Neasham, & Vineis 2006).

6. On the ethos of sanitary engineering and its relationship to germ theory, see Nash (2006). For the role of progressive social reformers in conducting urban surveys, see Sellers (1997).

7. Perhaps paradoxically, the successes of laboratory-based research on occupational health and illness contributed directly to the emergence of broader questions and concerns about the effects of environmental exposures on human health. Especially in the second half of the twentieth century, research on occupational health and illness "raised insistent questions about the interactions between the newly understood internal dynamics and the external environment," giving rise to the emergence of contemporary toxicology (Sellers 1997: 221).

8. According to Michaels (2008: 9), industry views "recall bias" in epidemiological studies, an aspect of exposure assessment, to be its "Achilles heel."

9. Epidemiologists report that even exposures that require individual choice and action, such as the number of alcoholic drinks one has per day, are difficult to ascertain (Interview 04).

10. I thank Ezra Susser for helping me to understand these dynamics; I could not have hoped for a more generous guide to the history of epidemiology.

11. I. Bernard Weinstein was a professor of medicine and of genetics at Columbia University and the Public Health Director of the Comprehensive Cancer Center. He is widely credited for recognizing that chemical contaminants in the environment would affect the human body at the molecular level. At URL: http://www.nytimes.com/2008/11/16/health/16weinstein.html.

12. At a workshop on the use of biomarkers in environmental health research, the U.S. National Academy of Sciences adopted this paradigm and expanded it to include a fourth category: "biomarkers of altered structure and function" (Vineis & Perera 2007: 1954).

13. Beginning in the 1970s, molecular biological techniques were commonly utilized by epidemiologists who studied particular vectors of disease. Indeed, the first use of the term "molecular epidemiology" was in a paper about influenza (Kilbourne 1973). In contrast, the molecular epidemiology pioneered by Perera and Weinstein uses molecular biomarkers as indicators signaling events in *human* biological systems or samples at the molecular or biochemical level (Perera and Weinstein 1999: 518).

14. Molecular processes that cause and/or are affected by mutagenesis— such as DNA damage, replication, recombination, and repair—are the foci of research on molecular mutagenesis. For important histories of this field, see Frickel (2004) and Lindee (1994).

15. A variety of biologic markers had been used for many years as tools in biomedical and epidemiologic research. For example, immunologists have long relied on white cell counts and antibody titers as indicators of infection (Schulte 1993: 19). Likewise, medical studies had begun to incorporate biochemical

markers as early as the 1930s (Kohler 1994). More recently, cardiovascular epidemiologists relied on blood pressure, serum cholesterol, and lipids as markers in their studies of cardiovascular disease (Shields & Harris 1991).

16. Molecular biomarkers of susceptibility include (1) markers pertaining to enzymes that increase or decrease the ability of a chemical to interact with DNA, RNA, or proteins; (2) markers of genetic differences in the capacity of cells to repair DNA damage caused by environmental insult; and (3) preexisting inherited genetic conditions that increase the risk of disease (Eubanks 1994).

17. The latency period varies across individuals and is sensitive to many parameters, including, for example, the type of exposure, the type of outcomes, nutrition, presence of comorbidity, and intervening events.

18. The *San Francisco Chronicle* initially reported that the study was conducted by the Agency for Toxic Substances and Disease Registry (ATSDR); this was incorrect (Lerner 2007). As will be described, at the request of the Midway Village residents, the ATSDR did review the study after it was completed; its assessment was quite critical.

19. Put differently, Midway Village may not be representative in a statistical sense. However, as Stinchcombe (2005) suggests, analysis can be advanced by sampling on the ends of a distribution, as well as at its center.

20. Because PG&E agreed to clean up the site, it ultimately was not remediated under the Superfund Program.

21. The EPA has classified seven PAH compounds as probable human carcinogens: benzo(a)anthracene, benzo(a)pyrene, benzo(b)fluoranthene, benzo(k) fluoranthene, chrysene, dibenz(a,h)anthracene, and indeno(1,2,3-cd)pyrene. This is largely consistent with the classification of PAHs by the International Agency for Research on Cancer (IARC). At URL: http://www.mass.gov/dep/toxics/pahs. htm. The State of California's Office of Environmental Health Hazard Assessment identifies eight additional PAHs as probable human carcinogens (Salocks 2006: 17).

22. According to the *San Francisco Examiner,* nearly 40% of 500 residents and former residents report serious illnesses, including breathing and digestive difficulties, reproductive and neurological problems, cancer, skin discoloration, and growths (Kay 1997b). There have been no peer-reviewed health assessments of Midway Village.

23. At the heart of any toxic tort action is the claim that a particular chemical substance or combination of substances has caused injury to the plaintiff. To make a persuasive case for compensation for injuries, therefore, the plaintiff must succeed in each of the following actions: (1) identify the harmful substance; (2) trace the pathway of exposure; (3) demonstrate that the exposure occurred at levels at which harm can result; (4) establish that the identified agent can cause injuries of the kind complained of; (5) rule out other possible causes of this injury (Jasanoff 1995: 119).

24.   These efforts focused on getting Section 8 vouchers for Midway Village tenants, so that they could move into private housing. However, given the extremely tight and expensive rental market in the San Francisco Bay area in 2000, this strategy was criticized by residents as ineffective (Pence 2000e).

25.   In fact that some soil samples were found to exceed EPA screening goals, resulting in the recommendation that the soil be removed by the state Department of Toxic Substances Control. The report also recommended further screening at nearby sites (Pence 2001a).

26.   The CEJAC review focuses primarily on issues of environmental justice and public participation at Midway Village. It includes, for example, a comparison of the cleanup of PAH contamination at Midway, where most of the residents are people of color, with the cleanup of similar pollution at Alhambra, near Los Angeles, where most of the residents are white. There are several differences between the two cleanup initiatives. First, in Alhambra, residents were relocated for six months while the cleanup took place, whereas at Midway there was no relocation during cleanup. Second, all the driveways, sidewalks, and patios at Alhambra were removed so that contaminated soil under them could be removed. Again, this did not take place at Midway. Third, an average of four to five feet of soil was removed at Alhambra, whereas two to five feet were removed at Midway. Fourth, soil from beneath the crawl space below the homes in Alhambra was removed, whereas the dirt beneath the living units at Midway remains untouched. In stark contrast to Midway Village, residents of Alhambra report being pleased with the remediation process in their community (Salocks 2006: 97).

27.   The committee received ten letters from Midway Village residents, describing the symptoms and illnesses that they and their family members have experiences while living at the site and requesting relocation. However, "because these letters contained personal health information" the OEHHA did not include the text of these letters in the final report (Salocks 2006: 70).

28.   These documents describe the analysis of soil, air, and groundwater samples collected at the site; the qualitative and statistical evaluation of the resulting data; the assessment of potential adverse effects on human health; and the effectiveness of the remedial strategies that were chosen to mitigate the risks to residents of the complex (Salocks 2006: 2).

29.   In her comments, Subra contends that neither assessment nor remediation at Midway Village have been adequate to protect the health of residents, noting particularly that "the remediation did not remove contaminated soils from under the housing units, buildings, sidewalks and streets" and "the use of only one set of a very few indoor air samples is inadequate on which to base the conclusion statement that PAHs in indoor air do not represent a significant health risk" (in Salocks 2006: 61–62).

30. The review committee notes in its response to the critical reviews of its draft report that the decision as to whether to conduct a community health assessment is beyond its purview and ultimately must be made by the Department of Health Services in consultation with officials from DTSC (Salocks 2006: 37).

31. At URL: http://www.nationalchildrensstudy.gov (accessed May 19, 2010).

32. Indeed, molecular epidemiology borrowed from the insights of a previous generation of environmental health scientists whose work established *environmental mutagenesis* as a legitimate independent object of scientific inquiry and of government regulation (Frickel 2004).

33. Monographs on the Evaluation of Carcinogenic Risks to Humans have been published by the IARC since 1971. They serve as a guide to regulatory and public health agencies. At URL: http://monographs.iarc.fr/(accessed May 16, 2010).

CHAPTER FIVE

1. Traditional sociological analyses recognize that diffusion often requires "translating concrete practices into abstractions for export and then unpacking the abstraction into a (suitably modified) concrete practice upon arrival" (Strang & Soule 1998: 277). From this perspective, translation occurs in the adopting context: "[P]ractices that travel from one site to another are modified and implemented *by adopters* in different ways so that they will blend into and fit the local social and institutional context" (Campbell 2005: 55, emphasis added). However, scholarship in STS shows that scientific practices do not "emerge fully formed from a politically and socially isolated world"; rather, scientists anticipate and act to address the concerns, standards, and requirements of those whom they wish to adopt their work (Keller 2009: 49).

2. In 2006, the NCT was "reconfigured" by the new leadership of the Institute. The core activities of the NCT have been maintained, however, in NIEHS laboratories focused on Environmental Genetics, Environmental Stress and Cancer, and Chemical Effects in Biological Systems (CEBS).

3. At URL: http://iccvam.niehs.nih.gov/about/about_ICCVAM.htm (accessed December 11, 2009).

4. A complete listing of the ICCVAM participating agencies is available at URL: http://iccvam.niehs.nih.gov/about/agencies/ni_AgRepS.htm (accessed December 11, 2009).

5. At URL: http://iccvam.niehs.nih.gov/about/about_ICCVAM.htm (accessed December 11, 2009). ICCVAM is an "internal governance unit" for toxicology testing (Fligstein & McAdam 2012: 78).

6. The National Toxicology Program Interagency Center for the Evaluation of Alternative Toxicological Methods (NICEATM) coordinates the activities that ICCVAM requires to evaluate and make recommendations regarding
new, revised, and alternative test methods. At URL: http://iccvam.niehs.nih
.gov/about/about_NICEATM.htm (accessed December 11, 2009).

7. To my surprise, scientists never referred to the Daubert standard in their
comments about relevance and reliability. Jasanoff (2005) provides an incisive
account of the Supreme Court case—*Daubert v. Merrell Dow Pharmaceuticals*—and
its legacy.

8. While NTP evaluation of a chemical typically includes a battery of long-
term and short-term tests, the gold standard for carcinogenicity testing is the
two-year rodent bioassay, a comprehensive evaluation that utilizes both sexes
of rats (Fischer 344/N) and mice (B6C3F1 hybrid) at three exposure levels, plus
untreated controls in groups of fifty animals.

9. I thank Adele Clarke for this helpful phrasing.

10. The National Toxicology Program reports have a blue cover and are
commonly referred to by insiders as "blue books".

11. These are known as Good Laboratory Practices (GLPs).

12. Drawing on Bowker and Star (2000), I understand standards to span
across communities of practice.

13. In fact, the future has already begun to arrive, as EPA's Office of Pesticide
Programs has received genomics articles as part of a data package submission for
a product registration. Further, research consortia in California and Washington
have begun to investigate genomics-based approaches to establishing water
quality standards (EPA 2004: 4–5).

14. On June 25, 2002, The EPA's Science Policy Council issued its *Interim Policy
on Genomics*, which was prepared for EPA staff and managers to communicate "to
interested parties external to EPA our initial thoughts concerning genomics . . . "
(EPA 2002). At URL: http://www.epa.gov/spc/pdfs/genomics.pdf (accessed
June 2, 2003). In December 2004, the EPA's Genomics Task Force Workgroup issued a white paper entitled *Potential Implications of Genomics for Regulatory and
Risk Assessment Applications at EPA*. At URL: http://www.epa.gov/osa/genomics
.htm (accessed September 13, 2009).

15. For an alternative perspective on the NAS, see Hilgartner (2000).

16. Significantly, one potential hot topic proposed by the NIEHS to be addressed by the NAS committee is, "Should the NRC report *Risk Assessment in the
Federal Government: Managing the Process*, the so-called Red Book, be updated to
address the new technologies and their potential impact on risk assessment?"
(NAS 2003: 3).

17. In conjunction with the formal NAS committee, the NIEHS organized a
"Federal Liaison Group," consisting of members of federal institutions that have

interests in toxicology and risk assessment. The Liaison Group is a critical component of the overall project because representatives of federal agencies (including the NIEHS) cannot be members of NAS committees.

18.   A complete list of workshop titles, presentations, and reports is available at URL: http://dels.nas.edu/emergingissues/events.shtml (accessed July 10, 2008).

19.   At URL: http://dels.nas.edu/envirohealth/ (accessed December 1, 2009).

20.   Specifically, topics "may include the use of information about gene-environment interactions in decisions regarding human health; the importance of environmentally mediated epigenetic modifications; use of mechanistic information about molecular pathways involved in toxicity; the impact of DNA repair processes on environmental health risks; application of technological advances in identifying chemical effects on gene, protein and metabolite expression; bioinformatics; computational and systems biology modeling; and methods for improving exposure assessment." At URL: http://dels.nas.edu/envirohealth/ (accessed 12/1/2009).

21.   As we will see, by 2010, EPA scientists were calling for a broader reimagining of the regulatory process (Firestone et al. 2010).

22.   The FDA and the EPA are the major federal regulatory agencies and "belong to a common social category" that promotes diffusion (Strang & Meyer 1993: 490). However, the agencies—and the situations they are charged to regulate—differ in multiple ways. First, at a technical level, drugs are a voluntary—and singular—exposure. As such, pharmacogenomics research generally investigates higher doses, focuses on a single chemical compound, and is more likely to include human subjects in research designs. Second, and related, the FDA is under more pressure to integrate genomic technologies into its procedures for regulatory review; compared to the chemical industry, the pharmaceutical industry has a greater interest—and has made a more significant investment—in genomic technologies (Interview P02). Third, the FDA relies heavily on data from industry in conducting regulatory reviews of pharmaceuticals. For all of these reasons, the extent to which the FDA is a helpful model for EPA in thinking about the role of genomic technologies in risk assessment appears to be an important domain for future social scientific research.

CHAPTER SIX

1.   These statistics are from 2000 and 2007, as noted. At URL: http://quick-facts.census.gov/qfd/states/28/28083.html (accessed June 15, 2009).

2.   In 2000, fewer than two-thirds of adults over 25 years of age in Leflore County had completed high school (compared to graduation rates of 73% in Mississippi and 80.4% nationally).

3.   Dr. Quinton also testified that the only other factor causing the children's impairments was "psychosocial issues," referring to how the children "had been nurtured" (Quinton 2005: 33). However, the defendants also raised the possibility that the plaintiffs had been exposed to lead at other locations (e.g., other residences or day care centers) (Byrd 2006b).

4.   Legal scholarship suggests that, although defendants are more likely to make a genetic argument to bolster their case, they are less likely to support their allegations with a genetic test than plaintiffs who raise such arguments (Hoffman & Rothenberg 2007: 869).

5.   The groundbreaking study of environmental racism, conducted under the auspices of the United Church of Christ, found that "those communities with the greatest percentages of minority residents had the most toxic waste facilities. . ." and that "percentage of minority population proved to be the strongest predictor of communities with the greatest number of waste facilities and the largest landfills" (Brown 1995: 17). A second major study found that "three of five Black and Hispanic individuals resided in a community with a CERCLIS [Super Fund] site" and that "three of five of the largest commercial hazardous waste landfills in the U.S., making up 40% of the nation's total capacity for hazardous waste landfills, were located in predominantly Black or Hispanic communities" (Brown 1995: 17). In the decades following these reports, studies of multiple regions of the United States and a variety of types of environmental hazards have found that that both race and class are significant determinates of proximity to known and prospective environmental hazards; further, they influence both the timing and extent of remediation actions (Brulle & Pellow 2006; IOM 1999).

6.   For example, the Southwest Network for Environmental and Economic Justice (SNEEJ) is "a regional, bi-national network founded in 1990 by representatives of 80 grassroots organizations based throughout the U.S. Southwest, California, and Northern Mexico" (in Faber & McCarthy 2001: 22).

7.   Examples include the Asian Pacific Environmental Network, Indigenous Environmental Network, and the Farmworker Network for Economic and Environmental Justice (Faber & McCarthy 2001: 9).

8.   Federal agencies vary widely in their responses to this order. For example, the definition of environmental justice offered by the Department of Health and Human Services focuses on the health *effects* of pollutants, whereas the Environmental Protection Agency's definition of environmental justice emphasizes equity in the *processes* through which risks are distributed. Likewise, there is variation in the enforcement of this order.

9.   Indeed, a single traditional environmental organization, the National Wildlife Federation, had an income of $82 million in 1998, about $39 million more than all combined foundation grants to the environmental justice movement that year (Faber & McCarthy 2001: 35).

10.   Eligible applicants for these grants are (1) a 501(c)(3) nonprofit organization as designated by the Internal Revenue Service; (2) a nonprofit organization, recognized by the state, territory, commonwealth, or tribe in which it is located; (3) a city, township, county government; *or* (4) a Native American tribal government (federally recognized) that is working in partnership with a disproportionately burdened community facing a specified public health issue. At URL: http://www.epa.gov/environmentaljustice/grants/ej-smgrants.html (accessed June 9, 2010).

11.   At URL: http://www.epa.gov/environmentaljustice/grants/ej-cps-grants.html (accessed June 9, 2010).

12.   Funding for EJ programs at both the EPA and the NIEHS has varied tremendously over time. For example, in 1995, the EPA awarded $3 million to 170 organizations through its Environmental Justice Small Grants Program; in 2004, it awarded $423,545 to just 17 organizations. According to the analysis of the NIEHS conducted by the Congressional Committee on Oversight and Government Reform (see Chapter 1), funding for the Environmental Justice: Partnerships for Communication Program was cut by 50% from Fiscal Year (FY) 2005 to FY 2007 (from $4,384,463 to $2,636,722), while funding for the CBPR Program was cut entirely in just three years (from $4 million in 2004 to $0 in 2007). At URL: http:// www.niehs.nih.gov/research/supported/dert/sphb/programs/justice/index .cfm (accessed September 15, 2012). During his presidential campaign, Barack Obama promised to reinvigorate federal environmental justice programs, including the EPA Office of Environmental Justice, and to expand the Environmental Justice Small Grants Program At URL: http://www.barackobama.com/pdf/ issues/EnvironmentFactSheet.pdf (accessed June 10, 2010).

13.   Collaborations may be undermined also by differences in power, access to financial resources, and race and class privileges among scientists and community members (Prakash 2004).

14.   For a review of "racial research" in science, see Tucker (1994).

15.   Reardon (2004) and Bliss (2012) provide compelling and contrasting accounts of the use of racial categories in genomics research.

16.   I am grateful to WEACT for allowing me to attend this symposium.

17.   "Field Notes, WEACT 2002" designates conversations and field notes taken during the conference, Human Genetics, Environment, and Communities of Color, organized by WEACT; it does not necessarily refer to notes taken in conversation with WEACT organizers or at the WEACT office. WEACT also published a conference summary, which I refer to as (WEACT 2002). I refer to the conference summary both as a means of triangulating the data I gathered and when I wish to quote directly from the statements published therein by conference participants.

18. WEACT remains at the forefront of the EJ movement's engagement with genetic and genomic research. At URL: http://www.weact.org/Events/PastEvents/GenesandJusticeACommunitySymposiumonHealth/tabid/224/Default.aspx (accessed June 10, 2009).

19. IPCB is a U.S.-based nonprofit organization created to assist Indigenous peoples in the protection of their genetic resources, knowledge, and cultural and human rights from the negative effects of biotechnology. At URL: http://www.ipcb.org/ (accessed October 2008).

20. See, for example, Patillo-McCoy and May 2000.

21. Advocates of genomics research have framed the same possibility in positive terms: "Perhaps awareness of genetic risk could galvanize genetic identity groups (those at risk) in ways that prompt community engagement and empowerment to influence social environmental exposures with an impact beyond those of current community organizing strategies?" (McBride et al. 2010: 558–559).

22. The Environmental Working Group (EWG), a U.S.-based environmental advocacy group, launched the Human Toxome Project (HTP) in order to define the "human toxome . . . the full scope of industrial pollution in humanity." At URL: http://www.ewg.org/sites/humantoxome/about/ (accessed February 4, 2009).

23. See, for example, Cells to Society (C2S): The Center on Social Disparities and Health at the Institute for Policy Research, at Northwestern University. At URL: http://www.northwestern.edu/ipr/c2s/ (accessed May 31, 2011) and the Institute of Medicine from Neurons to Neighborhoods Workshop. At URL: http://www.iom.edu/Activities/Children/Neuronstoneighborhoods/2010-OCT-28.aspx (accessed May 31, 2011).

CONCLUSION

1. Related, both symbolic interactionism and ANT are actively suspicious of any notion of "objective forces" or "social structure" as distinct from actors' direct interactions and personal connections (Bottero & Crossley 2011: 103).

2. On biomedicalization, see Clarke et al. 2003.

3. Of course, as a consequence of the relationship between environmental health research and environmental regulation, many conservative lawmakers would be happy to see significantly less federal support of environmental health institutions. On the whole, however, the EPA, rather than the NIEHS, has been the target of attacks by conservatives in Congress (Oreskes & Conway 2010: 147f). Between January and October 2011, Republicans in the U.S. House of Representatives brought to the floor no fewer than twelve bills designed to limit the

powers of the EPA. This analysis attends especially to how genetic and genomic technologies have been translated to the internal logic of the environmental health sciences (Martin 2003: 23).

4. Claims regarding genetic susceptibility have been especially central to the "doubt merchandizing" tactics of the tobacco industry (Oreskes & Conway 2010: 17, 28–29).

5. Fligstein and McAdam observe that the onset of contention is a field "typically starts with at least one collective actor defining some change in the field or external environment as constituting a significant new threat to, or opportunity for, the realization of group interests" (2011: 9). In this case, genetics was framed as both.

6. Indeed, industry is an "invisible interlocutor" in this analysis, as Stefan Timmermans helpfully pointed out. Although a few published reports on "industry perspectives" are available (Henry et al. 2002; Phillips 2008), this is important area for future research.

7. Public comments available at URL: http://www.regulations.gov/#!do cketDetail;dct=FR+PR+N+O+SR+PS;rpp=10;po=0;D=CDC-2011-0008 (accessed September 14, 2011).

8. In this same article, the authors noted that "as genomics continues to be applied in global healthcare settings, it must not be mistakenly used to divert attention and resources from the many non-genetic factors that contribute to health disparities, which would paradoxically exacerbate the problem" (Green et al. 2011: 210).

9. At URL: http://www.genome.gov/19518663 (accessed September 15, 2012).

10. At URL: https://www.phenx.org (accessed September 27, 2011).

11. PhenX engaged experts from relevant social, behavioral, and life sciences in establishing the measures in each domain. However, social scientists have expressed concern that research on gene-environment interaction tends to reduce complex social environments via "crude . . . indicators of social order" borrowed from epidemiological studies (Niewohner 2011: 294; see also Shim 2005).

12. Critics of this approach have highlighted the challenge of combining in one study "everything from sociological stresses to psychological stresses to chemical, physical, and biological stresses" and have suggested the importance— and complexity—of "a common metric" that can be used to make meaningful comparisons across these categories (Lioy, in Arnaud 2010).

13. Human genome research serves as not only a point of comparison for exposure scientists (e.g., as when they point out differential investments in technology development), but also a model. The exposome is proposed as a "complement" to the genome (Wild 2005), and advocates call for a Human Exposome

Project, similar in scope to the HGP. Further, they propose that the history of the HGP suggests that perceived barriers to technology development should not deter such efforts; the sequencing technologies that resulted in the successful completion of the HGP did not exist at the time it was launched.

14.   To date, there is tremendous variation in the breadth of exposures included in different scientists' visions of exposome research. A broad framework includes internal exposures (e.g., processes internal to the body such as metabolism, endogenous circulating hormones, body morphology, physical activity, gut microflora, inflammation, lipid peroxidation, oxidative stress and ageing), specific external exposures (e.g., radiation, infectious agents, chemical contaminants and environmental pollutants, diet, lifestyle factors (e.g. tobacco, alcohol), occupation and medical interventions), and wider social, economic and psychological influences on the individual (e.g., social capital, education, financial status, psychological and mental stress, urban–rural environment and climate) (Wild 2012: 24-25)[14]. More narrow definitions emphasize the internal consequences of individual behaviors, such as smoking and diet (Rappaport, et al. 2011)

15.   In contrast to exposomics, to date, EWAS research has focused on chemicals exposures—including nutritional supplements—and does not include measures of the social environment.

16.   Epigenetics actually appeared twice in the top five priorities, with number four being "Connecting environmental influences to disease through the study of epigenomics and epigenetic mechanisms . . . " At URL: http://www .niehs.nih.gov/about/od/strategicplan/stakeholder-community-workshop/ full-sp-workshop-report.pdf (accessed September 14, 2012).

17.   For a more detailed articulation of this argument, see Kuzawa and Sweet (2009).

18.   Niewohner notes that the researchers originally envisioned their research in terms of class but "switched to social position after sustained criticism from social scientists that class implies more than is measured with a few epidemiological variables of SES . . . " (2011: 286).

19.   Schnittker and MacLeod have critiqued the "downstream" focus of stress research (2005).

20.   I am indebted both to Everett Hughes (1971) and to Steve Epstein (2007) for modeling how sociological analyses can help us see that it "could be otherwise."

21.   In his seminal writing on fields, Bourdieu acknowledges that "outside forces" can shape their internal dynamics. However, he suggests further that the *scientific* field tends to be highly autonomous, with scientific production oriented wholly to other scientists whose primary goal is "recognition by the agent's

competitor peers" (Bourdieu 1975: 23). Indeed, part of the "specificity" of the scientific field, from this perspective, is its protection from political, economic, and religious concerns. Panofsky argues, "The fact that scientific truths are not simply determined by economic or political criteria means that the scientific field has a degree of autonomy from the economic and political fields" (2011: 298). However, in the case of the environmental health sciences, we see not a simple determination but 1) competition among scientific, economic, political, and social concerns in the formulation of risk assessment and regulation and (2) the powerful influence of political and economic interests in setting research agendas in the field.

22.   For example, "dependent ties to other strategic action fields that render a particular field vulnerable to exogenous shocks in 'turbulent times' tend to stabilize the field under ordinary circumstances" (Fligstein & McAdam 2012: 205).

23.   To be sure, I acknowledge that environmental health scientists in academic research centers engaged in "basic" research have more autonomy—and are less frequently called before the legislature or into courts—than scientists at the NTP. However, even scientists who are located in academic research centers maintain awareness of how policy debates will shape the trajectories of their research findings. For example, a molecular epidemiologist who studies gene-lead interaction told me with confidence that the policy impact of his research would be minimal unless the EPA or OSHA decides to "re-regulate" lead exposure. However, he continued, "that may change if we decide to go to electric vehicles or other kinds of vehicles" in which lead is used more extensively (Interview S11).

24.   Sismondo argues that, although the pharmaceutical industry may produce excellent scientific knowledge in clinical trials of its products, the fact that it dominates this form of knowledge production (in the United States) shapes the questions that are asked, the kinds of answers that are valued, and the direction of clinical and popular attention to certain medical conditions (2011). For a related analysis of pharmaceutical regulation, see Abraham and Ballinger (2011).

25.   Camic (2011) contends that this analytical approach is evident in Bourdieu's empirical studies of fields, despite and in contrast to his theoretical writings about the autonomy of the scientific field. It is also concordant with Bourdieu's criticism of sociological studies of science for "universalizing the particular case" and his emphasis on the importance of explicit analysis of the structural qualities of varied fields (1975: 29).

26.   These sorts of questions are also at the center of important new work on agnotology, or undone science (Proctor & Schiebinger 2008; Frickel, et al. 2010).

APPENDIX A

1. The initial stage of the research (2000–2003) was reviewed and approved by the Institutional Review Board of the University of California, San Francisco. The final year of the research was conducted under the purview of the IRB at the National Institutes of Health (which exempted the work from review). The oral history interviews that I conducted while at the NIH are in the public domain and available at the Office of NIH History.

2. Frickel (2011) similarly notes a "revolving door" of experts moving between academic, government, industry, and NGO jobs.

Glossary

American Chemistry Council	ACC
Cal/EPA Environmental Justice Advisory Committee	CEJAC
Centers for Disease Control and Prevention	CDC
Chemical Effects in Biological Systems (database)	CEBS
Department of Health and Human Services	DHHS
Department of Toxic Substances Control	DTSC
Environmental Protection Agency	EPA
Food and Drug Administration	FDA
Interagency Coordinating Committee on the Validation of Alternative Methods	ICCVAM
International Agency for Research on Cancer	IARC
Institute of Medicine	IOM

National Academy of Sciences   NAS

National Advisory Environmental Health Sciences Council   NAEHSC

National Cancer Institute   NCI

National Human Genome Research Institute   NHGRI

National Institute of Environmental Health Sciences   NIEHS

National Institutes of Health   NIH

NIH Chemical Genomics Center   NCGC

National Center for Toxicogenomics   NCT

National Research Council   NRC

National Toxicology Program   NTP

Office of Environmental Health Hazard Assessment   OEHHA

Toxicogenomics Research Consortium   TRC

TERMS[1]

Alcaptonuria   A relatively rare condition caused by an autosomal recessive
  genetic mutation that affects phenylalanine and tyrosine metabolism.

Carcinogen   An agent with the capacity to cause cancer in humans.

Carcinogenesis   The production of cancer; usually understood as a two-stage
  process, with initiation followed by promotion.

Chelation   A medical procedure using specific agents that bind with heavy
  metals as a means of removing them from the body.

Confocal microscopy   An imaging technique that allows scientists to "read"
  the fluorescence of samples spotted onto the array chips.

DNA   The chemical name for the molecule that carries genetic instructions
  in all living things.

DNA adduct   When a chemical or chemical metabolite covalently bonds to
  DNA, an adduct is formed. Adducts can interfere with the process of DNA
  replication, thereby causing mutations within a cell and initiating carcinogenesis.

DNA sequencing   A laboratory technique used to determine the exact sequence of bases (A, C, G, and T) in a DNA molecule.

Gene   The basic physical unit of inheritance. Genes are passed from parents
  to offspring and contain the information needed to specify traits.

---

1 Many of these definitions come from the NHGRI's online glossary at URL: http://
www.genome.gov/Glossary/index.cfm (accessed December 18, 2011).

Gene expression The process by which information from a gene is used to synthesize a product, such as a protein; it is central to how genetic information gives rise to bodily traits. Studying gene expression is a means of looking at how genes—in interaction with the environment and each other—generate specific phenotypes.

Genome The entire set of genetic instructions found in a cell. In humans, the genome consists of 23 pairs of chromosomes, found in the nucleus, as well as a small chromosome found in the cells' mitochondria. These chromosomes, taken together, contain approximately 3.1 billion bases of DNA sequence.

Genome-wide association studies (GWAS) An approach used in genetics research to associate specific genetic variations with particular diseases. The method involves scanning the genomes from many different people and looking for genetic markers that can be used to predict the presence of a disease.

Epigenetics An emerging field of science that studies heritable changes caused by the activation and deactivation of genes without any change in the underlying DNA sequence of the organism, but rather via methylation or histone modification. The word *epigenetics* is of Greek origin and literally means "over and above (epi) the genome."

Microarrays A developing technology used to study the expression of many genes at once. It involves placing thousands of gene sequences in known locations on a glass slide called a gene chip. A sample containing DNA or RNA is placed in contact with the gene chip. Complementary base pairing between the sample and the gene sequences on the chip produces light that is measured. Areas on the chip producing light identify genes that are expressed in the sample.

Mutagen A chemical or physical phenomenon, such as ionizing radiation, that promotes errors in DNA replication. Exposure to a mutagen can produce DNA mutations that cause or contribute to diseases such as cancer.

Mutagenesis The process by which genetic material, such as DNA and chromosomes, are changed (e.g., "mutated"). Environmental exposures are one mechanism of mutagenesis.

Northern blot A laboratory technique used to detect a specific RNA sequence in a blood or tissue sample. The sample RNA molecules are separated by size using gel electrophoresis. The RNA fragments are transferred out of the gel to the surface of a membrane. The membrane is exposed to a DNA probe labeled with a radioactive or chemical tag. If the probe binds to the membrane, then the complementary RNA sequence is present in the sample.

Polymerase chain reaction (PCR) A laboratory technique used to amplify DNA sequences. The method involves using short DNA sequences called "primers" to select the portion of the genome to be amplified. The temperature of the sample is repeatedly raised and lowered to help a DNA replication enzyme copy the target DNA sequence. The technique can produce a billion copies of the target sequence in just a few hours.

Polymorphism   One of two or more variants of a particular DNA sequence. The most common type of polymorphism involves variation at a single base pair. Polymorphisms can also be much larger in size and involve long stretches of DNA.

Single nucleotide polymorphism (SNP)   A polymorphism that involves variation at a single base pair.

Southern blot   A laboratory technique used to detect a specific DNA sequence in a blood or tissue sample. A restriction enzyme is used to cut a sample of DNA into fragments that are separated using gel electrophoresis. The DNA fragments are transferred out of the gel to the surface of a membrane. The membrane is exposed to a DNA probe labeled with a radioactive or chemical tag. If the probe binds to the membrane, then the probe sequence is present in the sample.

Xenobiotic   Chemical compounds that are foreign to a living organism.

Xenobiotic metabolism   The process by which compounds foreign to an organism are transformed and excreted.

References

Abbott, Andrew. 1988. *The System of Professions: An Essay on the Division of Expert Labor.* Chicago: University of Chicago Press.

Abraham, John, and Rachel Ballinger. 2011. "The Neoliberal Regulatory State, Industry Interests, and the Ideological Penetration of Scientific Knowledge: Deconstructing the Redefinition of Carcinogens in Pharmaceuticals." *Science, Technology, and Human Values* (online prepublication, accessed December 2, 2011).

Akaba, Azibuike. 2004. "Science as a Double-Edged Sword." *Race, Poverty, and the Environment* 11(2). Available at URL: http://urbanhabitat.org/node/10 (accessed July 3, 2012).

Albers, J. W. 1997. "Understanding Gene-Environment Interactions." *Environmental Health Perspectives* 105: 578–580.

Albert, Mathieu, and Daniel Kleinman. 2011. "Bringing Pierre Bourdieu to Science and Technology Studies." *Minerva* 49: 263–273.

Allen, Barbara. 2003. *Uneasy Alchemy: Citizens and Experts in Louisiana's Chemical Corridor Disputes.* Cambridge, MA: MIT Press.

————. 2004. "Shifting Boundary Work: Issues and Tensions in Environmental Health Science in the Case of Grand Bois, Louisiana." *Science as Culture* 13(4): 429–448.

Altman, Rebecca, Rachel Morello-Frosch, Julia Brody,Ruthann Rudel, Phil Brown, and Mara Averick. 2008. "Pollution Comes Home and Gets Personal: Women's Experience of Household Toxic Exposure" *Journal of Health and Social Behavior* 49(4): 417–435.

Ambrosone, Christine B., and Fred F. Kadlubar. 1997. "Toward an Integrated Approach to Molecular Epidemiology." *American Journal of Epidemiology* 146(11): 912–918.

Ames, B. N., W. E. Durston, E. Yamasaki, and F. D. Lee. 1973. "Carcinogens Are Mutagens: A Simple Test System Combining Liver Homogenates for Activation and Bacteria for Detection." *Proceedings of the National Academy of Sciences* 70(8): 2281–2285.

Arnaud, Celia Henry. 2010. "Exposing the Exposome." *Chemical & Engineering News* 88(33): 42–44.

Auyero, Javier, and Debora Swistun. 2009. *Flammable: Environmental Suffering in an Argentine Shantytown.* Oxford: Oxford University Press.

Balbus, John. 2008. "Toxicogenomics and the Public Interest: Technical and Sociopolitical Challenges." Pp. 46–56 in *Genomics and Environmental Regulation: Science, Ethics, and Law.* Edited by Richard R. Sharp, Gary Marchant, and Jamie A. Grodsky. Baltimore, MD: Johns Hopkins University Press.

Barrett, J. Carl. February 2004. Oral History Interview with the author. Office of NIH History.

Bartosiewicz, Matthew. M. Trounstine, David Barker, Richard Johnston, and Alan Buckpitt. 2000. "Development of a Toxicological Gene Array and Quantitative Assessment of This Technology." *Archives of Biochemistry and Biophysics* 376: 66–73.

Bartosiewicz, Matthew, Sharro Penn, and Alan Buckpitt. 2001. "Applications of Gene Arrays in Environmental Toxicology: Fingerprints of Gene Regulation Associated with Cadmium Chloride, Benzo(a)pyrene, and Trichloroethylene." *Environmental Health Perspectives* 109: 71–74.

Bearman, Peter. 2005. *Doormen.* Chicago: University of Chicago Press.

Beck, Ulrich. 1992. *Risk Society: Towards a New Modernity.* Thousand Oaks, CA: Sage.

Bell, Douglas A., Jack A. Taylor, David F. Paulson, Cary N. Robertson, James L. Mohler, and George W. Lucier. 1993. "Genetic Risk and Carcinogen Exposure: A Common Inherited Defect of the Carcinogen-Metabolism

Gene Glutathione-S Transferase M1 (GSTM1) That Increases Susceptibility to Bladder Cancer." *Journal of the National Cancer Institute* 85: 1159–11564.

Benford, Robert. 1993. "Frame Disputes Within the Nuclear Disarmament Movement." *Social Forces* 71: 677–702.

Benford, Robert D., and David A. Snow. 2000. "Framing Processes and Social Movements: An Overview and Assessment." *Annual Review of Sociology* 26: 611–639.

Beutler, E., R. J. Dern, and A. S. Alving. 1954. "The Hemolytic Effect of Primaquine: A Study of Primaquine Sensitive Erythrocytes." *Journal of Laboratory and Clinical Medicine* 44: 177–184.

Bliss, Catherine. 2012. *Race Decoded: The Genomic Fight for Social Justice.* Stanford, CA: Stanford University Press.

Bodmer, Walter, and Robin McKie. 1997. *The Book of Man: The Human Genome Project and the Quest to Discover Our Genetic Heritage.* Oxford: Oxford University Press.

Bookman, E. B., K. McAllister, E. Gillanders, K. Wanke, D. Balshaw, J. Rutter, J. Reedy, D. Shaughnessy, T. Agurs-Collins, D. Paltoo, A. Atienza ,L. Bierut, P. Kraft, M. D. Fallin, F. Perera, E. Turkheimer, J. Boardman, M. L. Marazita, S. M. Rappaport, E. Boerwinkle, S. J. Suomi, N. E. Caporaso, I. Hertz-Picciotto, K. C. Jacobson, W. L. Lowe, L. R. Goldman, P. Duggal, T. A. Manolio, E. D. Green, D. H. Olster, L. S. Birnbaum, for the NIH G × E Interplay Workshop participants. 2011. "Gene-Environment Interplay in Common Complex Diseases: Forging an Integrative Model—Recommendations from an NIH Workshop." *Genetic Epidemiology* 35(4): 217–225.

Bottero, Wendy, and Nick Crossley. 2011. "Worlds, Fields, and Networks: Becker, Bourdieu, and the Structures of Social Relations." *Cultural Sociology* 5(1): 99–119.

Bourdieu, Pierre. 1975. "The Specificity of the Scientific Field and the Social Conditions of the Progress of Reason." *Social Science Information* 14 (6): 19–47.

———. 1983. "The Field of Cultural Production, or: the Economic World Reversed." *Poetics* 12: 311–356.

———. 1996. *The Rules of Art: Genesis and Structure of the Literary Field.* Translated by S. Emanuel. Stanford, CA: Stanford University Press. Original edition, 1992.

———. 1998. Rethinking the State: Genesis and Structure of the Bureaucratic Field. In *Practical Reason: On the Theory of Action.* Edited by P. Bourdieu. Stanford, CA: Stanford University Press. Original edition, *Sociological Theory*, 1994.

———. 2004. *Science of Science and Reflexivity.* Chicago: University of Chicago Press.

Bourdieu, Pierre, and Loic Wacquant. 1992. *An Invitation to Reflexive Sociology.* Chicago, IL: University of Chicago Press.

Bowker, Geoffrey C., and Susan Leigh Star. 2000. *Sorting Things Out: Classification and Its Consequences.* Cambridge, MA: MIT Press.

Brandt, Allan M. 2007. *The Cigarette Century: The Rise, Fall, and Deadly Persistence of the Product That Defined America.* New York: Basic Books.

Brewer, George J. 1971. "Human Ecology, an Expanding Role for the Human Geneticist." *American Journal of Human Genetics* 23: 92–94.

Brown, Phil. 2007. *Toxic Exposures: Contested Illnesses and the Environmental Health Movement.* New York, NY: Columbia University Press.

Brown Phil, and Edwin J. Mikkelson. 1994. *No Safe Place: Toxic Waste, Leukemia, and Community Action.* Berkeley: University of California.

Brown, Phil Brian Mayer, and Meadow Linder. 2002. "Moving Further Upstream: From Toxics Reduction to the Precautionary Principle." *Public Health Reports* 117: 574–586.

Brown, Phil, Sabrina McCormick, Brian Mayer, Stephen Zavestoski, Rachel Morello-Frosch, Rebecca Gasior Altman, and Laura Senier. 2006. "A Lab of Our Own": Environmental Causation of Breast Cancer and Challenges to the Dominant Epidemiological Paradigm." *Science, Technology & Human Values* 31(September): 499–536.

Brulle, Robert J., and David Naguib Pellow. 2006. "Environmental Justice: Human Health and Environmental Inequalities." *Annual Review of Public Health* 27: 103–124.

Bryant, Bunyan, and Elaine Hockman. 2005. "A Brief Comparison of the Civil Rights Movement and the Environmental Justice Movement." Pp. 23–36 in *Power, Justice, and the Environment: A Critical Appraisal of the Environmental Justice Movement.* Edited by David Naguib Pellow and Robert J. Brulle. Cambridge, MA: MIT Press

Bullard, Robert D. 1994. *Unequal Protection: Environmental Justice and Communities of Color.* San Francisco: Sierra Club Books.

Burchiel, Scott W., Cindy M. Knall, John W. Davis, Richard S. Paules, Susan E. Boggs, and Cynthia A. Afshari,. 2001. "Analysis of Genetic and Epigenetic Mechanisms of Toxicity: Potential Roles of Toxicogenomics and Proteomics in Toxicology." *Toxicological Sciences* 59: 193–195.

Burawoy, Michael. 1999. "The Extended Case Method." *Sociological Theory,* 16(1): 4–33.

Burt, Ronald S. 1987. "Social Contagion and Innovation: Cohesion Versus Structural Equivalence." *American Journal of Sociology* 92(6): 1287–1335.

Byrd, Sheila. 2006a. "Gene Defense in Lead Paint Case Rankles." The Associated Press, July 13.

———. 2006b. "Mississippi Families Lose Suit Against Paint Maker." The Associated Press, August 7.

Cable, Sherry, Tamara Mix, and Donald Hasting. 2005. "Mission Impossible? Environmental Justice Movement Collaboration With Professional Environmentalists and with Academics." Pp. 55–76 in *Power, Justice, and the Environment: A Critical Appraisal of the Environmental Justice Movement.* Edited by David N. Pellow and Robert J. Brulle. Cambridge, MA: MIT Press.

Calabrese, Edward J. 1984. *Ecogenetics: Genetic Variation in Susceptibility to Environmental Agents.* New York: John Wiley & Sons.

———. 1986. "Ecogenetics: Historical Foundations and Current Status." *Journal of Occupational Medicine* 28(10): 1096–1102.

———. 1996. "Biochemical Individuality: The Next Generation." *Regulatory Toxicology and Pharmacology* 24: S58–S67.

Callon, Michel. 1995 "Four Models for the Dynamics of Science." Pp. 29–60 in *Handbook of Science and Technology Studies.* Edited by S. Jasanoff, G. E. Markle, J. C. Petersen, and T. J. Pinch. Thousand Oaks: Sage.

Camic, Charles. 2011. "Bourdieu's Cleft Sociology of Science." *Minerva* 49: 275–293.

Campbell, John L. 2005. "Where Do We Stand? Common Mechanisms in Organizations and Social Movements Research." Pp. 41–68 in *Social Movements and Organization Theory.* Edited by Gerald F. Davis, Doug McAdam, W. Richard Scott, and Mayer N. Zald. Cambridge: Cambridge University Press.

Capek, Stella M. 1993. "The 'Environmental Justice' Frame: A Conceptual Discussion and an Application." *Social Problems* 40(1): 5–24.

Carpenter, Daniel. 2010. *Reputation and Power: Organizational Image and Pharmaceutical Regulation at the FDA.* Princeton, NJ: Princeton University Press.

Carson, Paul E., C. Larkin Flanagan, C. E. Ickes, and Alf S. Alving. 1956. "Enzymatic Deficiency in Primaquine-Sensitive Erythrocytes." *Science* 124: 484.

Casper, Monica. 1998. *The Making of the Unborn Patient: A Social Anatomy of Fetal Surgery.* New Brunswick, NJ: Rutgers University Press.

Centers for Disease Control and Prevention (CDC). 1997. "Update: Blood Lead Levels. United States 1991–1994." *Morbidity and Mortality Weekly Report* 46(7): 141–146 and erratum in 46 (26): 607. U.S. Department of Health and Human Services. At URL: http://www.cdc.gov/mmwr/preview/mmwrhtml/mm4950a3.htm (accessed July 21, 2010).

————. 2003. *Surveillance for Elevated Blood Lead Levels Among Children—United States, 1997–2001.* Atlanta: U.S. Department of Health and Human Services. September 12, 2003 / 52(SS10);1–21. At URL: http: //www.cdc. gov/mmwr/preview/mmwrhtml/ss5210a1.htm (accessed July 21, 2010).

Charmaz, Kathy. 2006. *Constructing Grounded Theory: A Practical Guide Through Qualitative Analysis.* Thousand Oaks, CA: Sage.

Childs, Barton. 1970. "Sir Archibald Garrod's Conception of Chemical Individuality: A Modern Appreciation." *New England Journal of Medicine* 282(2): 71–77.

Christiani, David. 1996. "Utilization of Biomarker Data for Clinical and Environmental Intervention." *Environmental Health Perspectives* 104: 921–925.

Clarke, Adele E. 1998. *Disciplining Reproduction: Modernity, American Life Sciences, and the Problems of Sex.* Berkeley, CA: University of California Press.

————. 2005. *Situational Analysis: Grounded Theory After the Postmodern Turn.* Thousand Oaks, CA: Sage.

Clarke, Adele E., Janet K. Shim, Laura Mamo, Jennifer R. Fosket, and Jennifer R. Fishman. 2003. "Biomedicalization: Technoscientific Transformations of Health, Illness, and US Biomedicine." *American Sociological Review* 68: 161–194.

Collins, Francis S. 1999. "Shattuck lecture—Medical and Societal Consequences of the Human Genome Project." *New England Journal of Medicine* 341: 28–37.

————. 2001. "Contemplating the End of the Beginning." *Genome Research* 1(5): 641–643.

Collins, Francis S., Eric D. Green, Alan E. Guttmacher, and Mark S. Guyer. 2003. "A Vision for the Future of Genomics Research." *Nature* 422: 835–847.

Collins, Francis S., George M. Gray, and John R. Bucher. 2008. "Transforming Environmental Health Protection." *Science* 319(5865): 906–907.

Collins, Harry M. 1985. *Changing Order: Replication and Induction in Scientific Practice.* London: Sage.

Corburn, Jason. 2005. *Street Science: Community Knowledge and Environmental Health Justice.* Cambridge, MA: MIT Press.

————. 2009. *Toward the Healthy City: People, Places, and the Politics of Urban Planning.* Cambridge, MA: MIT Press.

Daniel, Mac. 2001. "Lead Paint Kills Young Refugee." *Boston Globe.* At URL: http: //www.ikecoalition.org/LSITF_News/NH_Guilty_Plea_Lead_ Poisoning.htm (accessed July 20, 2010).

Dean, Mitchell. 1999. *Governmentality: Power and Rule in Modern Society.* London: Sage.

de Chadarevian, Soraya, and Harmke Kamminga (Eds.). 1998. *Molecularizing Biology and Medicine: New Practices and Alliances, 1910s–1970s*. Amsterdam: Harwood Academic Publishers.

DeRisi, J., L. Penland, P. O. Brown, M. L. Bittner, P. S. Meltzer, P.S., et al. 1996. "Use of a cDNA Microarray to Analyse Gene Expression Patterns in Human Cancer." *Nature Genetics* 14: 457–460.

Dern, R. J., I. M. Weinstein, G. V. LeRoy, D. W. Talmage, and Alf S. Alving. 1954. "The Hemolytic Effect of Primaquine: The Localization of the Drug-Induced Hemolytic Effect in Primaquine-Sensitive Individuals." *Journal of Laboratory and Clinical Medicine* 43: 303–309.

DiMaggio, Paul, and W. Powell. 1983. "The Iron Cage Revisited: Institutional Isomorphism and Collective Rationality in Organizational Fields." *American Sociological Review* 48: 147–160

Duffy, John. 1992. *The Sanitarians: A History of American Public Health*. Urbana: University of Illinois Press.

Duneier, Mitchell. 1999. *Sidewalk*. New York: Farrar, Straus & Giroux.

Ellis, Juliet. 2004. "Burden of Proof: Using Research for Environmental Justice" *Race, Poverty, and the Environment* 11(2). Available at URL: http://urbanhabitat.org/node/54 (accessed July 3, 2012).

Engels, Friedrich. 1844 [1892]. *The Conditions of the Working Class in England*. London: Swan Sonnenschein & Co.

Environmental Health Perspectives (EHP). 1997. "Environmental Genome Project Advances." *Environmental Health Perspectives* 105: 1298.

Environmental Protection Agency (EPA). 2002. *Interim Genomics Policy*. Washington, DC: U.S. Environmental Protection Agency.

———. 2004. Genomics White Paper. EPA 100/B-04/002. Washington, DC: U.S. Environmental Protection Agency.

———. 2008. Memorandum of Understanding. Washington, DC: U.S. Environmental Protection Agency, National Center for Computational Toxicology.

Epstein, Steven. 1996. *Impure Science: AIDS, Activism, and the Politics of Knowledge*. Berkeley: University of California Press.

———. 2007. *Inclusion: The Politics of Difference in Medical Research*. Chicago, IL: University of Chicago Press.

Eubanks, M. 1994. "Biomarkers: The Clues to Genetic Susceptibility." *Environmental Health Perspectives* 102: 2–8.

Evans, David P. 1963. "Pharmacogenetics." *American Journal of Medicine* 34: 639–662.

Evans, Gary W., and Elyse Kantrowitz. 2002. "Socioeconomic Status and Health: The Potential Role of Environmental Risk Exposure." *Annual Review of Public Health* 23: 303–331.

Executive Order 12898. 1994 (February 11). Federal Actions to Address Environmental Justice in Minority Populations and Low Income Populations. Available at URL: http: //www.epa.gov/fedreg/eo/eo12898.htm (accessed June 10, 2010).

Faber, Daniel, and Deborah McCarthy, 2001. *Green of Another Color: Building Effective Partnerships Between Foundations and the Environmental Justice Movement.* Boston: Northeastern Environmental Justice Research Collaborative. Northeastern University.

Faustman Elaine M., and Gilbert S. Omenn. 1996. "Risk Assessment." Pp. 75–88 in *Casarett and Doull's Toxicology: The Basic Science of Poisons,* 5th ed. Edited by Curtis D. Klaassen. New York: McGraw-Hill.

Feero, W. G., A. E. Guttmacher, and F. S. Collins. 2008. "The Genome Gets Personal—Almost." *Journal of the American Medical Association* 299: 1351–1352.

Fielden, Mark R., and Tim R. Zacharewski. 2001. "Challenges and Limitations of Gene Expression Profiling in Mechanistic and Predictive Toxicology." *Toxicological Sciences* 60: 6–10.

Firestone, Michael, Robert Kavlock, Hal Zenich, Melissa Kramer, and the U.S. EPA Working Group on the Future of Toxicity Testing. "The U.S. Environmental Protection Agency Strategic Plan for Evaluating the Toxicity of Chemicals." *Journal of Toxicology and Environmental Health, Part B* 13: 139–162.

Fligstein, Neil. 2001. "Social Skill and the Theory of Fields." *Sociological Theory* 19: 105–125.

Fligstein, Neil, and Doug McAdam. 2011. "Toward a General Theory of Strategic Action Fields." *Sociological Theory* 29(1): 1–26.

———. 2012. *A Theory of Fields.* Oxford: Oxford University Press.

Food and Drug Administration (FDA). 2005. *Voluntary Genomic Data Submissions at the U.S. FDA.* Washington, DC: U.S. Food and Drug Administration.

Foucault, Michel. 1972/1980. *The Archeology of Knowledge and the Discourse on Language.* New York: Pantheon.

———. 1978/1990. *The History of Sexuality: An Introduction.* New York: Vintage Books.

Freese, Jeremy, and Sara Shostak. 2009. "Genetics and Social Inquiry." *Annual Review of Sociology* 35: 107–128.

Frickel, Scott. 2004. *Chemical Consequences: Environmental Mutagens, Scientist Activism, and the Rise of Genetic Toxicology*. New Brunswick, N.J.: Rutgers University Press.

———. 2011. "Who Are the Experts in Environmental Health Justice?" Pp. 21–40 in *Technoscience and Environmental Justice*. Edited by Gwen Ottinger and Benjamin Cohen. Cambridge, MA: MIT Press.

Frickel, Scott, Sahra Gibbon, Jeff Howard, Joanna Kempner, Gwen Ottinger, and David J. Hess. 2010. "Undone Science: Charting Social Movement and Civil Society Challenges to Research Agenda Setting." *Science, Technology, and Human Values* 35(4): 444–473.

Frickel, Scott and Neil Gross. 2005. "A General Theory of Scientific/Intellectual Movements." *American Sociological Review* 70: 204–232.

Frickel, Scott, and Kelly Moore (Eds.). 2006. *The New Political Sociology of Science: Institutions, Networks, and Power*. Madison: University of Wisconsin Press.

Fujimura, Joan. 1996. *Crafting Science: A Sociohistory of the Quest for the Genetics of Cancer*. Cambridge, MA: Harvard University Press.

Fullwiley, Duana. 2007. "The Molecularization of Race: Institutionalizing Racial Difference in Pharmacogenetics Practice." *Science as Culture* 16(1): 1–30.

Gallo, Michael A. 1996. "History and Scope of Toxicology." Pp. 4–11 in *Casarett & Doull's Toxicology: The Basic Science of Poisons*, 5th ed. Edited by Curtis D. Klaassen. New York: McGraw-Hill.

Garcia-Closas, M., K. T. Kelsey, X. Xu, and D.C. Christiani. 1997. "A Case-Control Study of Cytochrome P450 1A1, Glutathione S-Transferase M1, Cigarette Smoking and Lung Cancer Susceptibility." *Cancer Causes and Control* 8: 544–553.

Garrod, Archibald E. 1901. "About Alkaptonuria." *Lancet* 2: 1484–1486.

———. 1902. "The Incidence of Alkaptonuria: A Study in Chemical Individuality." *Lancet* 2: 1616–1630.

———.1909. *Inborn Errors of Metabolism*. London: Henry Frowde, Hodder and Staughton. Reissued as H. Harris (Ed.). 1963. *Garrod's Inborn Errors of Metabolism*. Oxford: Oxford University Press.

Gieryn, Thomas. 1999. *Cultural Boundaries of Science: Credibility on the Line*. Chicago: University of Chicago Press.

Glaser Barney G., and Anselm L. Strauss. 1967. *The Discovery of Grounded Theory*. Chicago, IL: Aldine.

Gordon, Jon W. 1989. "Transgenic Animals." *International Review of Cytology* 115: 171–229.

Gottweiss, Herbert M. 1995. *Governing Molecules: The Discursive Politics of Genetic Engineering in Europe and the United States* Cambridge, MA: MIT Press.

Granovetter, Mark S. 1973. "The Strength of Weak Ties." *American Journal of Sociology* 78(6): 1360–1380.

Green E. D., M. S. Guyer, and the National Human Genome Research Institute. 2011. "Charting a Course for Genomic Medicine from Base Pairs to Bedside." *Nature* 470: 204–213.

Grosse, Scott D., Thomas D. Matte, Joel Schwartz, and Richard J. Jackson. 2002. "Economic Gains Resulting from the Reduction in Children's Exposure to Lead in the United States." *Environmental Health Perspectives* 110 (61): 563–569.

Guengerich, F. P. 1998. "The Environmental Genome Project: Functional Analysis of Polymorphisms." *Environmental Health Perspectives* 106: 365–368.

Guttmacher, Alan E., and Francis S. Collins. 2003. "Welcome to the Genomics Era." *New England Journal of Medicine* 349(10): 996–998.

Haldane, J. B. S. 1938. *Heredity and Politics*. London: George Allen and Unwin.

Hamadeh, Hisham K., Pierre R. Bushel, Supriya Jayadev, Karla Martin, Olimpia DiSorbo, Lee Bennet, et al. 2002a. "Gene Expression Analysis Reveal Chemical Specific Profiles." *Toxicological Sciences* 67(2): 219–231.

———. 2002b. "Prediction of Compound Signature Using High Density Gene Expression Profiling." *Toxicological Sciences* 67(2): 232–240.

Hamlin, Christopher. 1992. "Predisposing Causes and Public Health in Early Nineteenth Century Medical Thought." *Social History of Medicine* 5(1): 43–70.

Harmon, Katherine. 2010. "Sequencing the 'Exposome': Researchers Take a Cue from Genomics to Decipher Environmental Exposure's Links to Disease." *Scientific American*. Available at URL: http://www.scientificamerican.com/article.cfm?id=environmental-exposure (accessed October 21, 2010).

Harper, Peter S. 2005. "William Bateson, Human Genetics and Medicine." *Human Genetics* 118: 141–151.

Hattis, Dale. 1996. "Variability in Susceptibility—How Big, How Often, for What Responses to What Agents?" *Environmental Toxicology and Pharmacology* 2: 135–145.

Haydu, Jeffrey. 1998. "Making Use of the Past: Time Periods as Cases to Compare and as Sequences of Problem Solving." *American Journal of Sociology* 104 (2): 339–371.

Hedgecoe, Adam M. 2001. "Schizophrenia and the Narrative of Enlightened Geneticization." *Social Studies of Science*, 31(6): 875–911.

———. 2004. *The Politics of Personalised Medicine: Pharmacogenetics in the Clinic.* Cambridge: Cambridge University Press.

Hedstrom, Peter, and Peter Bearman. 2009. "What is Analytical Sociology All About? An Introductory Essay." Pp. 3–24 in the *Oxford Handbook of Analytical Sociology.* Edited by Peter Hedstrom and Peter Bearman. Oxford: Oxford University Press.

Hemminki K., E. Grzybowska, P. Widlak and M. Chorazy. 1996. "DNA Adducts in Environmental, Occupational, and Life-Style Studies in Human Biomonitoring." *Acta Biochimica Polonica* 43: 305–312.

Henry, Carol, et al. 2002. "Use of Genomics in Toxicology and Epidemiology: Findings and Recommendations of a Workshop." *Environmental Health Perspectives* 110(10): 1047–1050.

Hess, David J. 2011. "Bourdieu and Science and Technology Studies: Toward a Reflexive Sociology." *Minerva* 49: 333–348.

Hilgartner, Stephen. 2000. *Science on Stage: Expert Advice as Public Drama.* Stanford, CA: Stanford University Press.

Hoffman, Diane E., and Karen H. Rothenberg. 2007. "Judging Genes: Implications of the Second Generation of Genetic Tests in the Courtroom." *Maryland Law Review* 66(4): 858–922.

Horwitz, Alan V. 2005. "Media Portrayals and Health Inequalities: A Case Study of Characterizations of Gene X Environment Interactions." *Journal of Gerontology* B 60: 48–52.

House, James S. 2002. "Understanding Social Factors and Inequalities in Health: 20th Century Progress and 21st Century Prospects." *Journal of Health and Social Behavior* 43(2): 125–142.

Hughes, Everett C. 1971. *The Sociological Eye.* Chicago: Aldine Atherton.

Institute of Medicine (IOM). 1999. *Toward Environmental Justice: Research, Education, and Health Policy Needs.* Washington, DC: National Academies Press.

———. 2006. *Genes, Behavior, and the Social Environment: Moving Beyond the Nature/Nurture Debate.* Washington, DC: National Academies Press.

———. 2010. *For the Public's Health: The Role of Measurement in Action and Accountability.* Washington, DC: National Academies Press.

Interagency Coordinating Committee on the Validation of Alternative Methods (ICCVAM). 1997. Validation and Regulatory Acceptance of Toxicological Test Methods. Research Triangle Park, NC: National Institute of Environmental Health Sciences. NIH Publication No: 97–3981. Available at URL: http://iccvam.niehs.nih.gov/docs/about_docs/validate.pdf (accessed 6/2/2011).

Jaroff, Leon. 1989. "The Gene Hunt." *Time Magazine.* 62–67 (March 20).

Jasanoff, Sheila. 1990. *The Fifth Branch: Science Advisors as Policymakers.* Cambridge, MA: Harvard University Press.

———. 1995. *Science at the Bar: Law, Science, and Technology in America.* Cambridge, MA: Harvard University Press.

———. 1996. "Science and Norms in International Environmental Regimes." Pp. 173–197 in *Earthly Goods: Environmental Change and Social Justice.* Edited by F. O. Hampson and J. Reppy. Ithaca, NY: Cornell University Press.

———. 2004. *States of Knowledge: The Co-Production of Science and the Social Order.* London: Taylor and Francis.

———. 2005. "Law's Knowledge: Science for Justice in Legal Settings." *American Journal of Public Health* 95(s1): 49–58.

Jasper, James. 2004. "A Strategic Approach to Collective Action: Looking for Agency in Social Movement Choices." *Mobilization* 9(1): 1–16.

Jensen, Wallace N. 1962. "Hereditary and Chemically Induced Anemia." *Archives of Environmental Health* 5: 212–216.

Kaiser, Jocelyn. 1997. "Environment Institute Lays Plans for Gene Hunt." *Science* 278(5338): 569–570.

———. 2011. "The Genome Project: What Will It Do as a Teenager?" *Science* 331: 660.

Kalow, Werner. 1962. *Pharmacogenetics.* Philadelphia, PA: Saunders.

———. 1968. "Drug Metabolism Enzymes. Pharmacogenetics in Animals and Man." *Annals of the New York Academy of Sciences* 151(2): 694–698.

———. 2001. Personal communication with the author.

Katznelson, Ira. 2003. "Periodization and Preferences: Reflections on Purposive Action in Comparative Historical Social Science." Pp. 270–301 in *Comparative Historical Analysis in the Social Sciences.* Edited by James Mahoney and Dietrich Rueschemeyer. Cambridge: Cambridge University Press.

Kay, Jane. 1997a. "Daly City Residents Living Atop Toxic Hot Spot." *San Francisco Examiner* April 27: A.

———. 1997b. "Daly City Toxics Lawsuit Tossed." *San Francisco Examiner* August 7: A.

Kay, Lily .E. 1993. *The Molecular Vision of Life: Caltech, the Rockefeller Foundation and the New Biology.* Oxford: Oxford University Press.

Keller, Ann. 2009. *Science in Environmental Policy: The Politics of Objective Advice.* Cambridge, MA: MIT Press.

Keller, Evelyn Fox. 2001. *The Century of the Gene*. Cambridge, MA: Harvard University Press.

Khoury, Muin J., Wylie Burke, and Elizabeth J. Thomson. 2000. *Genetics and Public Health in the 21st Century: Using Genetic Information to Improve Health and Prevent Disease*. Oxford: Oxford University Press.

Kilbourne, E. D. 1973. The Molecular Epidemiology of Influenza. *Journal of Infectious Diseases* 127: 478–487.

Kohler, Robert E. 1994. *Lords of the Fly: Drosophila Genetics and the Experimental Life*. Chicago: University of Chicago Press.

Krewski, Daniel, Melvin E. Andersen, Ellen Mantus, and Lauren Zeise. 2009. "Toxicity Testing in the 21st Century: Implications for Human Health Risk Assessment." *Risk Analysis* 29(4): 474–479.

Kuz, Martin. 2006. "What Lies Beneath," *San Francisco Weekly* December 20–26.

Kuzawa, Christopher W., and Elizabeth Sweet. "Epigenetics and The Embodiment of Race: Developmental Origins of US Racial Disparities in Cardiovascular Health." *American Journal of Human Biology* 21 (2009): 2-15.

Lamont, Michele. 2012. "How Has Bourdieu Been Good to Think With? The Case of the United States." *Sociological Forum* 27(1): 228–237.

Landecker, Hannah. 2011. "Food as Exposure: Nutritional Epigenetics and the New Metabolism." *BioSocieties* 6(2): 167–194.

Lanphear, B. P., T. D. Matte, J. Rogers, R. P. Clickner. B. Dietz, R. L. Bornschein, Succop, K. R. Mahaffey, S. Dixon. W. Galke. M. Rabinowitz, M. Farfel. C. Rohde. J. Schwartz , P. Ashley, and D. E. Jacobs. 1998. "The Contribution of Lead-Contaminated House Dust and Residential Soil to Children's Blood Lead Levels: A Pooled Analysis of 12 Epidemiological Studies." *Environmental Research* 79: 51–68.

Lanphear, B. P., R. Hornung, J. Khoury, K. Yolton, P. Baghurst, D. C. Bellinger, R. L. Canfield, K. N. Dietrich, R. Bornschein, T. Greene, S. J. Rothenberg, H. L. Needleman, L. Schnaas, G. Wasserman, J. Graziano, and R. Roberts. 2005. "Low-Level Environmental Lead Exposure and Children's Intellectual Function: An International Pooled Analysis." *Environmental Health Perspectives* 113(7): 894–899.

Larson, Shawna. 2004. "Science: More Harmful than Helpful?" *Race, Poverty, and the Environment* 11(2). Available at URL: http: //urbanhabitat.org/ node/11 (Accessed 7/3/2012)

Latour Bruno. 1987. *Science in Action: How to Follow Scientists and Engineers Through Society*. Cambridge, MA: Harvard University Press.

Lave, Rebecca. 2012. "Bridging Political Ecology and STS: A Field Analysis of the Rosgen Wars." *Annals of the Association of American Geographers* 102(2): 366–382.

Lerner, Steve. 2007. "Midway Village: Public Housing Built on Contaminated Soil." Available from the Collaborative on Health and the Environment, at URL: http://www.healthandenvironment.org/articles/homepage/789 (accessed August 14, 2010).

Lewis, Jack. 1985. "The Birth of EPA." *The EPA Journal.* Available at URL: http://www.epa.gov/aboutepa/history/topics/epa/15c.html (accessed June 4, 2009).

Lillienfield. D. E., and P. D. Stolley. 1994. *Foundations of Epidemiology.* Oxford: Oxford University Press.

Lindee, M. Susan. 1994. *Suffering Made Real: American Science and the Survivors at Hiroshima.* Chicago: University of Chicago Press.

———. 2005. *Moments of Truth in Genetic Medicine.* Baltimore, MD: The Johns Hopkins University Press.

Link, Bruce G. and Jo C. Phelan. 1995. "Social Conditions as Fundamental Causes of Disease." *Journal of Health and Social Behavior,* 35 (supplement): 80-94.

Lippman, Abby J. 1991. "Prenatal Genetic Testing and Screening: Constructing Needs and Reinforcing Inequities." *American Journal of Law and Medicine* 17: 15–50.

Livingston, Robert J., Andrew Von Niederhausern, Anil G. Jegga, Dana C. Crawford, Christopher S. Carlson, Mark J. Rieder, Sivakumar Gowrisankar, Bruce J. Aronow, Robert B. Weiss, and Deborah A. Nickerson. 2004. "Pattern of Sequence Variation Across 213 Environmental Response Genes." *Genome Research* 14: 1821–1831.

Lobenhofer, Edward K., Poerre R. Bushel, Cynthia A. Afshari, and Hisham K. Hamadeh. 2001. "Progress in the Application of DNA Microarrays." *Environmental Health Perspectives* 109: 881–891.

Loffredo, Christoper A., Ellen K. Silbergeld, and Mark Parascandola. 1998. "The Environmental Genome Project: Suggestions and Concerns." *Environmental Health Perspectives* 106(8): 368.

Loomis, D., and S. W. Wing. 1990. "Is Molecular Epidemiology a Germ Theory for the End of the Twentieth Century?" *International Journal of Epidemiology* 19: 1–3.

Lord, Peter B. 2001. "No Sanctuary in America." *Providence Journal.* At URL: http://www.projo.com/cgi-bin/include.pl/extra/lead/stories/day3.htm (accessed July 21, 2010).

Lovett, Richard A. 2000. 'Toxicologists Brace for Genomics Revolution." *Science* 289: 536–537.

MacArthur, D. 2008. "Why Do Genome Wide Scans Fail?" *Genetic Future*. Available at URL: http://www.genetic-future.com/2008/03/why-do-genome-wide-scans-fail.html (accessed September 18, 2011).

Mancinelli, Laviero, Maureen Cronin, and Wolfgang Sadee. 2000. "Pharmacogenomics: The Promise of Personalized Medicine." *AAPS PharmSci* 2(1): art. 4. Available at URL: http: //www.aapsj.org/view.asp?artpps020104.

Manuel, John. 1996. "Environment, Genes, and Cancer." *Environmental Health Perspectives* 104(3): 256–258.

Marcus, George. 1995/1998. "Ethnography in/of the World System: The Emergence of Multi-Sited Ethnography." Pp. 79–104 in *Ethnography Through Thick and Thin*. Princeton, NJ: Princeton University Press.

Markowitz, Gerald, and David Rosner. 2002. *Deceit and Denial: The Deadly Politics of Industrial Pollution*. Berkeley: University of California Press.

Martin, John Levi. 2003. "What Is Field Theory?" *American Journal of Sociology* 109: 1–49.

McBride, Colleen, Deborah Bowen, Lawrence Brody, et al. 2010. "Future Health Applications of Genomics: Priorities for Communication, Behavioral, and Social Sciences Research." *American Journal of Preventive Medicine* 38(5): 556–561.

Medina, Daniel, Robert Ullrich, Raymond Meyn, Roger Wiseman,and Larry Donehower. 2002. "Environmental Carcinogens and p53 Tumor-Suppressor Gene Interactions in a Transgenic Mouse Model for Mammary Carcinogenesis." *Environmental and Molecular Mutagenesis* 39(2/3): 178–183.

Meier, Hans. 1963. *Experimental Pharmacogenetics: Physiopathology of Heredity and Pharmacologic Responses*. New York: Academic Press.

Mendelsohn, J. Andrew. 2001. "Medicine and the Making of Bodily Inequality in Twentieth Century Europe." *Heredity and Infection: The History of Disease Transmission*. Edited by J. P. Gaudilliere and Ilana Lowy. London: Routledge.

Merrill, Ray M. 2008. *Environmental Epidemiology: Principles and Methods*. Sudbury, MA: Jones & Bartlett.

Mialet, Helene. 2003. "The Righteous Wrath of Pierre Bourdieu." *Social Studies of Science* 33: 613–621.

Michaels, David. 2008. *Doubt Is Their Product: How Industry's Assault on Science Threatens Your Health*. Oxford: Oxford University Press.

Mittman, G., M. Murphy, C. and Sellers. (Eds). 2004. "Landscapes of Exposure; Knowledge and Illness in Modern Environments." *Osiris*, 19.

Montague, Peter. 2004. "Deceptive Science: The Problem with Risk Assessment." *Race, Poverty, and the Environment* 11(2). Available at URL: http://urbanhabitat.org/node/1557 (accessed July 3, 2012).

Moore, Kelly. 2008. *Disrupting Science: Social Movements, American Scientists, and the Politics of the Military, 1945–1975.* Princeton, NJ: Princeton University Press.

Morales, Jose. 2002. *Genomic Justice: Environmental Justice Biotechnology Policy.* Working Paper. New York: Public Interest Biotechnology.

Morris Julian (Ed.). 2000. *Rethinking Risk and the Precautionary Principle.* Boston: Butterworth- Heinemann.

Motulsky, Arno. 1957. "Drug Reactions, Enzymes, and Biochemical Genetics." *Journal of the American Medical Association* 165: 835–837.

———. 2002. "The Work of Joseph Adams and Archibald Garrod: Posible Examples of Prematurity in Human Genetics." In *Prematurity and Scientific Discovery.* Edited by E. B. Hook. Berkeley: University of California Press.

Mountain, John T. 1963. "Detecting Hypersusceptibility to Toxic Substances." *Archives of Environmental Health* 6: 357–365.

Murphy, Michelle. 2006. *Sick Building Syndrome and the Problem of Uncertainty: Environmental Politics, Technoscience, and Women Workers.* Durham, NC: Duke University Press.

Nash, Linda. 2006. *Inescapable Ecologies: A History of Environment, Disease, and Knowledge.* Berkeley: University of California Press.

National Academy of Sciences (NAS). 1973/1975. *Principles for Evaluating Chemicals in the Environment.* Presented at Principles for Evaluating Chemicals in the Environment, Washington, DC.

———. 1993. *Measuring Lead Exposure in Infants, Children, and Other Sensitive Populations.* Washington, DC: Committee on Measuring Lead in Critical Populations, Board on Environmental Studies and Toxicology, Commission on Life Sciences, National Academy of Sciences, National Academy Press.

———. 2003. "Emerging Issues in the Environmental Health Sciences', National Academy of Sciences Newsletter, volumes 1–6.

National Center for Toxicogenomics (NCT). 2002. *Using Global Genomic Expression Technology to Create a Knowledge Base for Protecting Human Health.* Research Triangle Park, NC: National Institute of Environmental Health Sciences.

National Institute of Environmental Health Sciences (NIEHS). 1997. *Environmental Genome Project Symposium.* Bethesda, MD: National Institutes of Health.

————. 2000a. Environmental Genome Project Overview. Available at URL: http: //www.nieh.nih.gov/egp.htm.

————. 2000b. Toxicogenomics Research and Environmental Health Introduction. Available at URL: http: www.niehs.nih.gov/dert/ programs.htm.

————. 2006 (February 8). "Two NIH Initiatives Launch Intensive Efforts to Determine Genetic and Environmental Roots of Common Diseases." Press Release 06-03. National Institutes of Health.

National Institutes of Health (NIH) 2008. "NIH Collaborates with EPA to Improve the Safety Testing of Chemicals." Available at URL: http: //www .nih.gov/news/health/feb2008/nhgri-14.htm.

National Research Council (NRC). 1983. *Risk Assessment in the Federal Government: Managing the Process*. Washington, DC: National Academy Press.

————. 2007a. *Applications of Toxicogenomics Technologies to Predictive Toxicology and Risk Assessment*. Washington, DC: National Academy Press.

————. 2007b. *Toxicity Testing in the 21st Century: A Vision and a Strategy*. Washington, DC: National Academy Press.

National Toxicology Program (NTP). 1984. *Report of the NTP Ad Hoc Panel on Chemical Carcinogenesis Testing and Evaluation*. Available at URL: http: // ntp.niehs.nih.gov/?objectid=720164F2-BDB7-CEBA-F5C6A2E21851F0C4 q (accessed March 18, 2011).

————. 2002. *Current Directions and Evolving Strategies*. Washington, DC: Department of Health and Human Services.

Nelkin Dorothy. 1989. "Testing in the Workplace: Predicting Performance and Health." Pp. 75–105 in *Dangerous Diagnostics: The Social Power of Biological Information*. Edited by Dorothy Nelkin and Lawrence Tancredi. New York: Basic Books.

Nelkin, Dorothy, and M. Susan Lindee. 2004. *The DNA Mystique: The Gene as a Cultural Icon*. Ann Arbor: University of Michigan Press.

Niewohner, Jorg. 2011. "Epigenetics: Embedded Bodies and the Molecularisation of Biography and Milieu." *BioSocieties* 6(3): 279–298.

Nuwaysir, Emile F., Michael Bittner, Jeffrey Trent, J. Carl Barrett, and Cynthia A. Afshari. 1999. "Microarrays and Toxicology: The Advent of Toxicogenomics." *Molecular Carcinogenesis* 241: 153–159.

Olden, Kenneth. 2001. Fiscal Year 2002. NIEHS Statement for House and Senate Appropriations Subcommittees. April 4.

————. 2002. "New Opportunities in Toxicology in the Post-Genomic Era." *Drug Discovery Today* 7: 273–276.

Olden, Kenneth. July 2004. Oral History Interview with the author. Office of NIH History.

————. 2000. "Public Health Genetics: An Emerging Interdisciplinary Field for the Post- Genomic Era." *Annual Review of Public Health* 21, 1–13.

Olden, Kenneth, Nicholas Freudenberg, Jennifer Dowd, and Alexandra E. Shields. 2011. "Discovering How Environmental Exposures Alter Genes Could Lead to New Treatments for Chronic Illnesses." *Health Affairs* 30(5): 833–841.

Olden, Kenneth, and Janet Guthrie. 2001. "Genomics: Implications for Toxicology." *Mutation Research* 473: 3–10.

Olden, Kenneth, Janet Guthrie, and Sheila Newton. 2001. "A Bold New Direction for Environmental Health Research." *American Journal of Public Health* 91(12): 1964–1967.

Olden, Kenneth, and Sandra. L. White. 2005. "Health-Related Disparities: Influence of Environmental Factors." *Medical Clinics of North America* 89(4): 721–738.

Olden, Kenneth, and Samuel Wilson. 2000. "Environmental Health and Genomics: Visions and Implications." *Nature Reviews Genetics* 1: 149–153.

Omenn, Gilbert S., and H. V. Gelboin. 1983. *Genetic Variability in Responses to Chemical Exposure*. New York: Cold Spring Harbor Laboratory.

Ong, Elisa K., and Stanton A. Glantz. 2001. "Constructing 'Sound Science' and 'Good Epidemiology': Tobacco, Lawyers, and Public Relations Firms." *American Journal of Public Health* 91: 1749–1755.

Oreskes, Naomi, and Erik M. Conway. 2010. *Merchants of Doubt: How a Handful of Scientists Obscured the Truth on Issues from Tobacco Smoke to Global Warming*. New York: Bloomsbury Press.

Ottinger, Gwen. 2009. "Epistemic Fencelines: Air Monitoring Instruments and Expert-Residents Boundaries." *Spontaneous Generations: A Journal for the History and Philosophy of Science* 3(1): 55–67.

Ottinger, Gwen, and Benjamin Cohen. 2011. *Technoscience and Environmental Justice*. Cambridge, MA: MIT Press.

Ottman, Ruth. 1995. "Gene-Environment Interaction and Public Health." *American Journal of Human Genetics* 56: 821–823.

Paneth, Nigel. Peter Vinten-Johansen, Howard Brody, and Michael Rip. 1998. "A Rivalry of Foulness: Official and Unofficial Investigations of the London Cholera Epidemic of 1854." *American Journal of Public Health* 88: 1545–1553.

Panofsky, Aaron. 2011. "Field Analysis and Interdisciplinary Science: Scientific Capital Exchange in Behavior Genetics." *Minerva* 49: 295–316.

Parodi, Alessandra, David Neasham, and Paolo Vineis. 2006. "Environment, Population, and Biology: A Short History of Modern Epidemiology." *Perspectives in Biology and Medicine* 49(3): 357–368.

Patel, Chirag J., Jayanta Bhattacharya, and Atul J. Butte. 2010. "An Environment-Wide Association Study (EWAS) on Type 2 Diabetes Mellitus." PLOS 5(5): 1–10.

Pattillo-McCoy, Mary and Rueben Buford May. 2000. "Do You See What I See? Examining a Collaborative Ethnography." *Qualitative Inquiry.* 6:1 (65–87).

Paules, Richard. S., Raymond Tennant, J. Carl Barrett, and George W. Lucier. 1999. "Bringing Genomics into Risk Analysis: The Promises and Problems." *Risk Policy Report* 17(September): 30–33.

Pellow, David Naguib, and Robert J. Brulle (Eds.). 2005. *Power, Justice, and the Environment: A Critical Appraisal of the Environmental Justice Movement.* Cambridge, MA: MIT Press.

Pence, Angelica. 2000a. "Gene Defects for Neighbors of Toxic Site." *San Francisco Chronicle* January 19: A-1.

———. 2000b. "Living on Toxic Ground." *San Francisco Chronicle* January 20: A-1.

———. 2000c. "Relocation Sought for Tenants Living on Toxic Ground: Federal Emergency Funds Requested." *San Francisco Chronicle* January 26: A-13.

———. 2000d. "Neighbors of Toxic Site Plan to Sue." *San Francisco Chronicle* February 18: A-21.

———. 2000e. "HUD Proposal to Move Tenants from Toxic Site." *San Francisco Chronicle* March 14: A-13.

———. 2000f. "Daly City Soil Tests Begin, But Method Is Already Criticized." *San Francisco Chronicle* June 27: A-21.

———. 2001a. "Midway Tests Show No Threat From Toxics." *San Francisco Chronicle* February 3: A-2.

———. 2001b. "Tenants Blast State Toxics Agency." *San Francisco Chronicle* February 28: A-15.

Pennie, William D., Jonathan D. Tugwood, Gerry J. Oliver, and Ian Kimber. 2000. "The Principles and Practice of Toxigenomics: Applications and Opportunities." *Toxicological Sciences* 54: 277–283.

Perera, Frederica P. 1987. "Molecular Cancer Epidemiology: A New Tool in Cancer Prevention." *Journal of the National Cancer Institute* 78: 887–898.

———. 1997. "Environment and Cancer: Who Are Susceptible?" *Science* 278: 1068–1073.

————. 2000. "Molecular Epidemiology: On the Path to Prevention?" *Journal of the National Cancer Institute* 92: 602–612.

Perera, Frederica P., and I. Bernard Weinstein. 1982. "Molecular Epidemiology and Carcinogen-DNA Adduct Detection: New Approaches to Studies of Human Cancer Causation." *Journal of Chronic Disease* 35: 581–600.

————. 2000. "Molecular Epidemiology: Recent Advances and Future Directions." *Carcinogenesis* 213: 517–524..

Pescosolido, Bernice. 2006. "Of Pride and Prejudice: The Role of Sociology and Social Networks in Integrating the Health Sciences." *Journal of Health and Social Behavior* 47: 189–208.

Petersen, Alan, and Deborah Lupton. 1996. *The New Public Health: Health and Self in the Age of Risk.* London: Sage.

Phillips, Richard D. 2008. "Applications of Genomics for Health and Environmental Safety of Chemicals: An Industry Perspective." Pp. 35–45 in *Genomics and Environmental Regulation: Science, Ethics, and Law.* Edited by Richard R. Sharp, Gary Marchant, and Jamie A. Grodsky. Baltimore, MD: Johns Hopkins University Press.

Pierson, Paul. 2000. "Increasing Returns, Path Dependence, and the Study of Politics." *The American Political Science Review* 94(2): 251–267.

Pirkle, J. L., D. J. Brody, E. W. Gunter, R. A. Kramer, D. C. Paschal, K. M. Flegal, and T. D. Matte. 1994. "The Decline in Blood Lead Levels in the United States. The National Health and Nutrition Examination Surveys." *JAMA* 272: 284–291.

Pirkle, J.L., R. B. Kaufmann, D. J. Brody, T. Hickman, E. W. Gunter, and D. C. Paschal. 1998. "Exposure of the U.S. Population to Lead, 1991–1994." *Environmental Health Perspectives* 106: 745–750.

Pollack, Andrew. 2000. "DNA Chip May Help Usher in a New Era of Product Testing." *New York Times,* November 28.

Polletta, Francesca. 1998. "'It Was Like a Fever…': Narrative and Identity in Social Protest." *Social Problems* 45: 137–159.

Prakash, Swati. 2004. "Power, Privilege, and Participation." *Race, Poverty, and the Environment* 11(2). Available at URL: http://urbanhabitat.org/node/155 (accessed July 3, 2012).

Pritchard, John B., John E. French, Barbara J. Davis, and Joseph K. Haseman. 2003. "The Role of Transgenic Mouse Models in Carcinogen Identification." *Environmental Health Perspectives* 111(4): 444–454.

Proctor, Robert N. 1995. *Cancer Wars: How Politics Shapes What We Know and Don't Know About Cancer.* New York: Basic Books.

Proctor, Robert N., and Londa Schiebinger (Eds.). 2008. *Agnotology: The Making and Unmaking of Ignorance*. Stanford, CA: Stanford University Press.

Puga Alvaro, J. Micka, C. Chang, H. Liang, and Daniel W. Nebert. 1996. "Role of Molecular Biology in Risk Assessment." *Advances in Experimental Medicine and Biology* 387: 395–404.

Quinton, Barbara A. 2005a. Report to the Court. Case: *Tamiko Jones, et al. v. NL Industries, et al.*

———. 2005b. Transcript of the Testimony of Barbara A. Quinton. December 12, 2005 (printed December 19, 2005). Case: *Tamiko Jones, et al. v. NL Industries, et al.*

Rabin, Richard. 1989. "Warnings Unheeded: A History of Child Lead Poisoning." *American Journal of Public Health* 79(1): 1668–1674.

Rabinow, Paul, and Nikolas Rose. 2006. "Biopower Today." *BioSocieties* 1: 195–217.

Ragin, Charles C. 1992. *What is a Case?: Exploring the Foundations of Social Inquiry*. Cambridge: Cambridge University Press.

Rapp, Rayna. 1999. *Testing Women/Testing the Fetus: The Social Impact of Amniocentesis in America*. New York: Routledge.

Rappaport, Stephen. 2010. "Frontiers in Exposure Science." Presentation to the Committee on Emerging Science for Environmental Health Decisions. Washington, DC: National Academy of Sciences.

Rappaport, Stephen M., and Martyn T. Smith. 2010. "Environment and Disease Risks." *Science*, 330(6003): 460–461.

Rappaport, Stephen M., He Li, Hasmik Grigoryan, William E. Funk, and Evan R. Williams. 2011. "Adductomics: Characterizing Exposures to Reactive Electrophiles." *Toxicology Letters* 213: 83–90.

Reardon, Jenny. 2004. *Race to the Finish: Identity and Governance in an Age of Genomics*. Princeton, NJ: Princeton University Press.

Research Triangle Institute (RTI). 1965. "Recommendations for the Development and Operation of a National Environmental Health Sciences Center." Department of Health, Education, and Welfare, U.S. Public Health Service, Bureau of State Services (Environmental Health). Research Triangle Park, NC.

Revkin, Andrew C. 2001. "Scientists Track Contaminants, Inside the Body and Out." *New York Times* May 15.

Rockett, J. C., and D. J. Dix. 1999. "Application of DNA Arrays to Toxicology." *Environmental Health Perspectives* 107: 681–685.

Rose Nikolas. 2001. "The Politics of Life Itself." *Theory, Culture, and Society* 18: 1–30.

_____. 2007. *The Politics of Life Itself: Biomedicine, Power, and Subjectivity in the Twenty-First Century*. Princeton, NJ: Princeton University Press.

Rosen, George. 1993 (1958). *A History of Public Health* (expanded edition). Baltimore, MD: Johns Hopkins University Press.

Rosenberg, Charles. (2007) *Our Present Complaint: American Medicine, Then and Now.* Baltimore, MD: Johns Hopkins University Press.

Rushefsky, Mark. 1986. *Making Cancer Policy*. Albany, NY: SUNY Press.

Salocks, Charles. 2006. "Review of the 2001 Investigation and Cleanup of Midway Village Residential Complex in Daly City, California." Review draft, February 2006.

Schena, M., D. Shalon, R. W. Davies, and P. O. Brown. 1995. "Quantitative Monitoring of Gene Expression with a Complementary DNA Microarray." *Science* 270: 476–470.

Schettler, Ted, Gina Solomon, Maria Valenti, and Annette Huddle. 2000. *Generations at Risk: Reproductive Health and the Environment*. Cambridge, MA: MIT Press.

Schmidt, C. W. 2002. "Toxicogenomics: An Emerging Discipline." *Environmental Health Perspectives* 110: 750–756.

_____. 2009. "Tox21: New Dimensions of Toxicity Testing." *Environmental Health Perspectives* 117(8): 348–353.

Schneiberg, Marc, and Elisabeth S. Clemens. 2006. "The Typical Tools for the Job: Research Strategies in Institutional Analysis." *Sociological Theory* 24(3): 195–228.

Schnittker, Jason, and Jane D. McLeod. 2005. "The Social Psychology of Health Disparities." *Annual Review of Sociology* 31: 75–103.

Schulte, P. A. 1993. "A Conceptual and Historical Framework for Molecular Epidemiology." In *Molecular Epidemiology: Principles and Practices*. Edited by Paul. A .Schulte and Frederica P. Perera. San Diego, CA: Academic Press.

Schulte, Paul A., and Frederica P. Perera (Eds.). 1993. *Molecular Epidemiology: Principles and Practices*. San Diego, CA: Academic Press.

Schwartz, B. S., B. K. Lee, G. S. Lee, W. F. Stewart, D. Simon, K. Kelsey, and A. C. Todd. 2000. "Associations of Blood Lead, Dimercaptosuccinic Acid-Chelatable Lead, and Tibia Lead with Polymorphisms in the Vitamin D Receptor and [delta]-Aminolevulinic Acid Dehydratase Genes." *Environmental Health Perspectives* 108(10): 949–954.

Schwartz, David, and Francis S. Collins. 2007. "Environmental Biology and Human Disease." *Science* 316: 695–696.

Schwetz, Bern A. 2001. "Toxicology at the Food and Drug Administration: New Century, New Challenges." *International Journal of Toxicology* 20: 3–8.

Sellers, Christopher. 1997. *Hazards of the Job: From Industrial Disease to Environmental Health Science.* Chapel Hill, NC: University of North Carolina Press.

Shapin, Steven. 1994. *A Social History of Truth.* Chicago, IL: University of Chicago Press.

————. 2008. *The Scientific Life: A Moral History of a Late Modern Vocation.* Chicago, IL: University of Chicago Press.

Sharp, Richard R., Gary Marchant, and Jamie A. Grodsky (Eds). 2008. *Genomics and Environmental Regulation: Science, Ethics, and Law.* Baltimore, MD: Johns Hopkins University Press.

Shelby, Michael. April 2004. Oral History Interview with the author. Office of NIH History.

Shepard, Peggy, Mary E. Northridge, Swati Prakash, and Gabriel Stover. 2002. "Advancing Environmental Justice Through Community Based Participatory Research." *Environmental Health Perspectives* 110(Supplement 2): 139–140.

Shields, P. G., and C. C. Harris. 1991. "Molecular Epidemiology and the Genetics of Environmental Cancer." *Journal of the American Medical Association* 246: 681–687.

Shim, Janet K. 2005. "Constructing 'Race' across the Science-Lay Divide: Racial Formation in the Epidemiology and Experience of Cardiovascular Disease." *Social Studies of Science* 35(3): 405–436.

Shostak, Sara. 2007. "Translation at Work: Genetically Modified Mouse Models and Molecularization in the Environmental Health Sciences." *Science, Technology, and Human Values* 32(3): 315–338.

Shostak, Sara, Jeremy Freese, Bruce G. Link, and Jo C. Phelan. 2009. "The Politics of the Gene: Social Status and Beliefs about Genetics for Individual Outcomes." *Social Psychology Quarterly* 72(1): 77–93.

Simmons, Beth A., Frank Dobbin, and Geoffrey Garrett (Eds.). 2008. *The Global Diffusion of Markets and Democracy.* Cambridge: Cambridge University Press.

Simmons, Trinia, and Christopher J. Portier. 2002. "Toxicogenomics: The New Frontier in Risk Analysis." *Carcinogenesis* 23: 903–905.

Sismondo, Sergio. 2011. "Bourdieu's Rationalist Science of Science: Some Promises and Limitations." *Cultural Sociology.* Available at URL: http://cus.sagepub.com/content/5/1/83.abstract?rss=1 (accessed Decmber 1, 2011.)

Sloan, Phillip R. 2000. "Completing the Tree of Descartes." Pp. 1–25 in *Controlling Our Destinies: Historical, Philosophical, Ethical, and Theological Perspectives on the Human Genome Project.* Edited by Phillip R. Sloan. Notre Dame, IN: University of Notre Dame Press.

Smith E. 1996. "Variability in Toxic Response—Relevance to Chemical Safety and Risk Assessment at the Global Level." *Environmental Toxicology and Pharmacology* 2: 85–88.

Smith, Lewis L. 2001. "Key Challenges for Toxicologists in the 21st Century." *Trends in Pharmacological Sciences* 22: 281–285.

Smith, R. J. 1979. "NCI Bioassays Yield a Trail of Blunders." *Science* 204(4399): 1287–1292.

Smith, Martyn, and Stephen Rappaport. 2009. "Building Exposure Biology Centers to Put the E into 'G × E' Interaction Studies." *Environmental Health Perspectives* 117(8): 334–335.

Smithies, O., and H. S. Kim. 1994. "Targeted Gene Duplication and Disruption for Analyzing Quantitative Genetic Traits in Mice." *Proceedings of the National Academy of Science of the United States of America* 91 (9): 3612–3615.

Snow, David A., E. Burke Rochford, Steven K. Worden, and Robert D. Benford. 1986. "Frame Alignment Processes, Micromobilization, and Movement Participation." *American Sociological Review* 51: 464–481.

Steingraber, S. 2003. *Having Faith.* Cambridge, MA: Perseus.

Stinchcombe, Arthur. 2005. *The Logic of Social Research.* Chicago, IL: University of Chicago Press.

Stokinger, Herbert E. 1962. "New Concepts and Future Trends in Toxicology." *Journal of the American Industrial Hygiene Association* 23: 9–19.

Stokinger, H. E., J. T. Mountain, and L. D. Scheel. 1968. "Pharmacogenetics in the Detection of the Hypersusceptible Worker." *Annals of the New York Academy of Sciences* 151: 968–976.

Stone, Deborah A. 1989. "Causal Stories and the Formation of Policy Agendas." *Political Science Quarterly* 104(2): 281–300.

———. 2001. *Policy Paradox: The Art of Political Decision Making,* 3rd ed. New York: W. W. Norton.

Stone, R. 1993. "Ken Olden Heals NIEHS's 'Split Brain.'" *Science* 259(5100): 1398–1399.

Strang, David, and John W. Meyer. 1993. "Institutional Conditions for Diffusion." *Theory and Society* 22: 487–511.

Strang, David, and Sarah A. Soule. 1998. "Diffusion in Organizations and Social Movements: From Hybrid Corn to Poison Pills." *Annual Review of Sociology* 24: 265–290.

Sturdy, Steve. 1998. "Reflections: Molecularization, Standardization and the History of Science." Pp. 273–293 in *Molecularizing Biology and Medicine:*

New Practices and Alliances, 1910s–1970s. Edited by Soraya de Chadarevian and Harmke Kamminga. Amsterdam: Harwood Academic Publishers.

Susser, Mervyn, and Ezra Susser. 1996a. "Choosing a Future for Epidemiology I: Eras and Paradigms." *American Journal of Public Health* 86: 668–673.

———. 1996b. "Choosing a Future for Epidemiology II. From Black Box to Chinese Boxes and Eco-Epidemiology." *American Journal of Public Health* 86: 874–877.

Szasz, A. 2007. *Shopping Our Way to Safety: How We Changed from Protecting the Environment to Protecting Ourselves*. Minneapolis: University of Minnesota Press.

Sze, Julie. 2007. *Noxious New York: The Racial Politics of Urban Health and Environmental Justice*. Cambridge, MA: MIT Press.

Sze, Julie, and Swati Prakash. 2004. "Human Genetics, Environment, and Communities of Color: Ethical and Social Implications." *Environmental Health Perspectives*. 112(6): 740–745.

Tamiko Jones, et al. v. NL Industries, et al. (Civil Action No. 4: 03CV229).

Tarlov, Alvin R., George J. Brewer, Paul E. Carson, and Alf S. Alving. 1962. "Primaquine Sensitivity: Glucose-6-Phosphate Dehydrogenase Deficiency: An Inborn Error of Metabolism of Medical and Biological Significance." *Archives of Internal Medicine* 109: 209–234.

Tennant, Raymond W. 2001. "The National Center for Toxicogenomics: Using New Technologies to Inform Mechanistic Toxicology." *Environmental Health Perspectives* 110: A8–A10.

Tennant, Raymond W. November 2004. Oral History Interview, with the author. Office of NIH History.

Tennant, Raymond W., John E. French, and Judson W. Spalding. 1995. "Identifying Chemical Carcinogens and Assessing Potential Risk in Short-Term Bioassays Using Transgenic Mouse Models." *Environmental Health Perspectives* 103(10): 942–950.

Tennant, R. W., B. H. Margolin, M. D., Shelby, E. Zeiger, J. K. Haseman, J. Spalding. W. Caspary, M. Resnick. S. Stasiewicz. and B. Anderson. 1987. "Prediction of Chemical Carcinogenicity in Rodents from in Vitro Genetic Toxicity Assays." *Science:* 236(4804): 933–941.

Thelen, Kathleen. 1999. "Historical Institutionalism in Comparative Politics." *Annual Review of Political Science* 2: 369–404.

———. 2003. "How Institutions Evolve: Insights from Comparative Historical Analysis." Pp. 208–240 in *Comparative Historical Analysis in the Social Sciences*. Edited by James Mahoney and Dietrich Rueschemeyer. Cambridge: Cambridge University Press.

Tickner. J. (Ed.) 2003. *Precaution, Environmental Science, and Preventive Public Policy.* Washington, DC: Island Press.

Timmermans, Stefan, and Marc Berg. 1997. "Standardization in Action: Achieving Local Universality Through Medical Protocols." *Social Studies of Science* 27: 273–305.

Timmermans, Stefan, and Iddo Tavory. 2007. "Advancing Ethnographic Research Through Grounded Theory Practice." Pp. 493–512 in *The Sage Handbook of Grounded Theory.* Edited by Anthony Bryant and Kathy Charmaz. Thousand Oaks, CA: Sage.

Tolich, Martin. 2004. "Internal Confidentiality: When Confidentiality Assurances Fail Relational Informants." *Qualitative Sociology.* 27(1): 101–106.

Tucker, William H. 1994. *The Science and Politics of Racial Research.* Champagne-Urbana: University of Illinois Press.

Ugolini, Donatella, Ricardo Puntoni, Frederica P. Perera, Paul A. Schulte, and Stefano Bonassi. 2007. "A Bibliometric Analysis of Scientific Production in Cancer Molecular Epidemiology." *Carcinogenesis* 28(8): 1774–1779.

United States Government Printing Office (US GPO). 2007. "Will NIEHS' New Priorities Protect Public Health?" Hearing Before the Subcommittee on Domestic Policy of the Committee on Oversight and Government Reform, House of Representatives, One Hundred Tenth Congress, First Session. Available at URL: http: //www.gpoaccess.gov/congress/index.html (accessed June 2, 2010).

Vineis, Paolo. 2004. "A Self-fulfilling Prophecy: Are We Underestimating the Role of the Environment in Gene–Environment Interaction Research?" *International Journal of Epidemiology* 33: 945–946.

Vineis, Paolo, and Frederica P. Perera. 2000. "DNA Adducts as Markers of Exposure to Carcinogens and Risk of Cancer." *International Journal of Cancer* 88: 325–328.

———. 2007. "Molecular Epidemiology and Biomarkers in Etiologic Cancer Research: The New in Light of the Old." *Cancer Epidemiology Biomarkers & Prevention* 16(10): 1954–1965.

Vogel, Sarah A. 2008. "From 'the Dose Makes the Poison' to 'the Timing Makes the Poison': Conceptualizing Risk in the Synthetic Age." *Environmental History* 13(4). Available at URL: http: //www.environmentalhistory.net/articles/13-4_Vogel.htm (accessed October 12, 2011).

Wakefield, Jerome C. 2002. "Environmental Genome Project: Focusing on Differences to Understand the Whole." *Environmental Health Perspectives* 110: 756–760.

Waller, John C. 2002a. "The Illusion of an Explanation: The Concept of Hereditary Disease, 1770–1870." *Journal of the History of Medicine and Allied Science* 57(4): 410–488.

Waller, John C. 2002b. "Ideas of Heredity, Reproduction, and Eugenics in Britain, 1800–1875." *Studies in the History and Philosophy of Biology and Biomedical Science* 32: 457–489.

Weber, Wendell, W. 2001. "The Legacy of Pharmacogenetics and Potential Applications." *Mutation Research* 479: 1–18.

West Harlem Environmental Action (WEACT). 2002. *Human Genetics, Environment, and Communities of Color: Ethical and Social Implications.* New York.

Whyatt, Robin M, Regina M. Santella, Wieslaw Jedrychowski, Seymour J. Garte, Douglas A. Bell, Ruth Ottman, Alicja Gladek-Yarborough, Greg Cosma, Tie-Lan Young, Thomas B. Cooper, Mary C. Randall, David K. Manchester, Frederica P. Perera. 1998. "Relationship Between Ambient Air Pollution and DNA Damage in Polish Mothers and Newborns." *Environmental Health Perspectives* 106(S3): 821–826.

Wild, Christopher P. 2005. "Complementing the Genome with an 'Exposome': "Challenge of Environmental Exposure Measurement in Molecular Epidemiology." *Cancer Epidemiology, Biomarkers & Prevention* 14(8): 1847–1850.

———. 2012. "The Exposome: From Concept to Utility." *International Journal of Epidemiology* 4: 24–32

Williams, David R. 2005. "The Health of U.S. Racial and Ethnic Populations." *Journal of Gerontology: Social Sciences* 60B: 53–62.

Williams, David R., and Selina A. Mohammed. 2009. "Discrimination and Racial Disparities in Health: Evidence and Needed Research." *Journal of Behavioral Medicine* 32: 20–47.

Williams, David R., Selina A. Mohammed, Jacinta Leavell, and Chiquita Collins. 2010. "Race, Socioeconomic Status, and Health: Complexities, Ongoing Challenges, and Research Opportunities." *Annals of the New York Academy of Sciences* 1186: 69–101.

Wilson, Samuel H., and Kenneth Olden. 2004. "The Environmental Genome Project: Phase I and Beyond." *Molecular Interventions* 4(3): 147–156.

Weisburger, Elizabeth K. 1983. "History of the Bioassay Program of the National Cancer Institute." *Progress in Experimental Tumor Research* 26: 187–201.

Zavon, Mitchell R. 1962. "Modern Concepts of Diagnosis and Treatment in Occupational Medicine." *Journal of the American Industrial Hygiene Association* 23: 30–36.

Index